Just Because You're Depressed Doesn't Mean You Have Depression
Or
Depression Is a Symptom
Not a Disease
So
Find the Cause
Fix the Problem

By
Mary Ann Block, DO

Block System Books are published by
The Block System
1750 Norwood Drive
Hurst, Texas 76054

The Block System and The Block System logo
Reg. US Pat. & Off.
First Printing:
Printed in the United States of America

This publication is designed to provide accurate and authoritative information with regard to the subject matter covered. The purchase of this publication does not create a doctor-patient relationship between the purchaser and the author, nor should the information contained in this book be considered specific medical advice with respect to a specific patient and/or a specific condition. In the event the purchaser desires to obtain specific medical advice or other information concerning a specific person, condition or situation, the services of a competent professional should be sought.

The author and publisher specifically disclaim any liability, loss, or risk, personal or otherwise, that is or may be incurred as a consequence, directly or indirectly, of the use and application of any of the information contained in this book.

Dedicated to Kim, Chris and Larry

Who might be alive today if they had not taken

antidepressants.

Remembering Lee Hyman,

my friend and editor

A special thank you
to Rana K. Williamson, PhD
for her valuable assistance and
exceptional editorial contribution to this book.

Just Because You're Depressed

WARNING

Never rapidly discontinue the use of antidepressants. Stopping an antidepressant should be done slowly and under a doctor's supervision.

Introduction

I write this book with the same purpose with which I approached all my books: to share information with others. When prescription drugs intended to heal my daughter actually made her more ill, I made a life-changing decision. I went to medical school, at age 39, to learn what doctors learn. I didn't want what happened to my daughter to happen to anyone else I love.

After medical school, I went into practice to directly share my knowledge with others who also wished to protect their families. My mantra became, "No one should have to go to medical school to protect their loved ones." Still I am thankful, every day, that I became a physician.

The resources I found following my mother's diagnosis of "terminal," metastatic lung cancer helped her to recover completely. At M.D. Anderson Cancer Center doctors gave her two months to live. Four months into her treatment, she was declared "cancer free." That was 17 years ago. Today my mother is 91 years old.

At 92 my father's cardiologist sent him home to die of fluid in the heart and lungs. Knowing the limits of medicine, I called an osteopathic cardiologist, who removed the fluid from both areas and recommended cardiac rehabilitation exercises. My father became healthier than ever. He passed away at the age of 98 with a strong mind and a strong heart.

Each day patients tell me stories that make me realize how fortunate I am to have the knowledge I have gained. In many instances the previous medical treatments my patients received might have produced better results had a physical exam or lab work been done or the side effects of a given drug been acknowledged.

As a physician I try to give the patient all the information and let them make an educated decision about their care. Regardless of what their decision may be, I believe it is critical that they be fully informed.

In the past fifteen years, especially with the introduction of Health Maintenance Organizations (HMOs), major changes have occurred in the practice of medicine that do not always benefit the patient. Reduced fees prevent doctors from spending more than five to seven minutes with a patient. In that short amount of time a physician simply cannot explore the possible underlying causes of a medical problem. All the doctor can do is listen to the chief complaint and write a prescription. Quick. Easy. Cheap. In my opinion, that's just not good medicine.

Online sources indicate the top 10 drugs sold in 2005 in the United States were:

1.	Lexapro	6.	Phentermine
2.	Paxil	7.	Neurontin
3.	Zoloft	8.	Vioxx
4.	Wellbutrin	9.	Effexor
5.	Xanax	10.	Bextra

Six of the ten are psychiatric drugs used to treat depression. This confirms to me that doctors are not taking time to evaluate patients and are just prescribing antidepressants instead.

When the patient identifies depression as their chief complaint, a brief examination won't suffice to get to the real root of the problem. A doctor in a hurry may resort to simply writing a prescription for an "easy fix" drug you don't really need. Antidepressant medications are plentiful – quick, easy, cheap. But just because you're depressed doesn't mean you have depression. And just because the doctor wrote the prescription, doesn't mean you actually need it.

Everyone deserves to have a physician who will take a thorough history, do a complete physical exam, and look for the true underlying medical cause of a person's symptoms. No one should accept a doctor who just listens to your chief complaint and hands you a prescription. Everyone deserves more.

Life Is Not a Psychiatric Disorder
Mary Ann Block, DO

Giving birth should be happy,
but you don't feel that way.
Postpartum depression is what people say.
You're prescribed antidepressants called SSRI
Which keep you even, and won't let you cry.
After giving birth you may feel sad and alone.
But it's not psychiatric, just messed up hormones.

When kids wiggle in school and just can't sit still,
They're given a psych label and most often, a pill.
It's much more than that or can't you see?
Their diets are terrible, they're not ADHD.
We could fix the problem. Instead of a drug,
Try changing their diets, then, give them a hug.

The stages of grief number five, they say.
And you can't get through them
in a quicker way.
It starts with denial and we must walk, not run.
Through all the others till acceptance comes.
When someone dies we need to say good-bye.
Not cover our grief with another SSRI.

Emotions are normal, sometimes we feel bad.
Some days we are happy, on others we're sad.
But the ups and downs are better by far,
When put all together, they make up who we are.
From the time you are born,
you have stress, pain and strife.
But it's not psychiatric,
it's just a condition called life.

Section I - The Depression Industry-What You Need To Know To Be Informed

Ch. 1: Life Is Not a Psychiatric Disorder or *Just Because You're Depressed, Doesn't Mean You Have Depression*

Ch. 2: The Diagnostic and Statistical Manual or *Just Because It's Written Down, Doesn't Make It True*

Ch. 3: Understanding the Medical System or *If All You Have Is A Prescription Pad, Everyone Gets A Drug*

Section II - Find the Cause — Fix the Problem — What They Don't Want You To Know

Ch. 4: The Thyroid and Adrenal Glands or *If Their Not Working, You're Not Working*

Ch. 5: It's Not Depression, It's De' Hormones or *Are Your Hormones Driving You Crazy?*

Ch. 6: Magnesium or *A Simple Nutrient Could Save Your Life*

Ch. 7: Allergies or *Depression Is Nothing to Sneeze At*

Ch. 8: Drug Side Effects or *What You Don't Know Can Hurt You*

Appendix I
Protocol and Resources or *Find the Cause, Fix the Problem*

Appendix II
Cardiac and Nervous System Side Effects of Antidepressants or These Drugs Can Kill

Appendix III
Definitions of medical terms

IMPORTANT

Never rapidly discontinue the use of antidepressants. Stopping an antidepressant should always be done slowly and under a doctor's supervision.

Section I
The Depression Industry
What You Need To Know To Be Informed

Chapter 1
Life Is Not a Psychiatric Disorder
or
Just Because You're Depressed,
Doesn't Mean You Have Depression

For Carolyn* it began after the birth of her second child. With two babies only 16 months apart, she began to feel like her life was out of control. "Here I was trying to care for a two-month-old and an 18-month-old and every day felt like a struggle," she recalled. "I didn't feel depressed exactly. It was more like I was overwhelmed with too much on my plate. It all made me feel a bit stressed and anxious." (*Names have been changed to protect the privacy of the patients.*)

After struggling to get through the next four months, she decided to tell her internist how she was feeling. He immediately recommended that she go on Prozac, telling her she had post-partum depression. "At first I resisted because of the stigma that is attached to this diagnosis, but after some thought, I realized I needed help and nothing else was being offered," she explained. So she decided to try the drug.

Carolyn felt better at first but she never got enough relief from the drug. So a few months later, after the holidays when her youngest was a year old, she decided to stop the drug cold turkey. "No one had been monitoring me or telling me that you need to wean yourself slowly from the drug," she said. "They never did any kind of follow up." But the symptoms became more pronounced, so she went back on the drug. When she saw her obstetrician a few months later, she told him about her symptoms. He recommended that she double the dose of Prozac from 10 mg. to 20 mg. in order to get more relief.

3

After eight months on the higher dose, she decided to get pregnant with her third baby so she went off the drug again. And again, not knowing the dangers, she did it cold turkey. When she was five months into her pregnancy, she told her obstetrician that she was concerned about a repeat of the post-partum depression. He recommended that she go back on the 20 mg. of Prozac at that point so that the drug would have more than the four to six weeks to build up in her system. She delivered and nursed her baby while taking the drug. From that point, Carolyn stayed on the drug for two years although occasionally trying to stop it saying that "the drug was not working very well." Even though the drug was less effective, she seemed to feel worse when she wasn't taking it.

When she told her obstetrician that she was not happy being on Prozac and that she had concerns about the stigma associated with it, the doctor tried to prescribe her something else. But it was just Prozac under a different name, Sarafem. When Carolyn told him she knew that the drug was Prozac, he admitted to trying to disguise it, telling her that she was smarter than the average patient.

He offered no other options. Consequently, the same cycle continued to repeat itself. Carolyn would take the drug for awhile, decide to go off it, but return to the prescription when the absence of the drug made her feel worse. Then a series of frightening and debilitating symptoms began to take control of her life. First, she began experiencing horrific joint pain. Her hip hurt the worst with the pain shooting down her entire leg. She couldn't sleep and could barely sit in a chair for more than a few minutes at a time. She saw an orthopedic specialist. Carolyn told the doctor that she was taking Prozac during her first appointment. The specialist did an MRI and x-rays but could find nothing wrong with her.

When she started experiencing chest pains, she rushed to the emergency room. After a frightening wait, the doctor reported that she had pleurisy not a cardiac-related problem. She was relieved. But the ER doctor was deeply concerned about the results of her blood test which showed that her liver enzymes were elevated, often an indicator for some serious conditions.

Carolyn was aware of the problem. Blood tests showing elevated enzymes began during her last pregnancy. Her obstetrician sent her to a specialist in diseases of the digestive tract. Carolyn told this specialist that she was taking the Prozac. He was concerned she had hepatitis but tests were negative. He recommended that she come back after the pregnancy to do some additional tests, which she did. He ran various tests including an MRI and sonograms of her liver. All tests had come back negative. The doctor wanted to do a liver biopsy but, because it is such an invasive procedure, he decided to watch her for a while first. She saw the doctor every six weeks. During that time her enzyme levels bounced from normal to elevated levels with each test. At the same time, Carolyn was going on and off Prozac trying to stop the drug. The doctor called her condition a mystery.

Carolyn suffered great fatigue and does not know how she managed to take care of her children. "I never felt good. I couldn't get out of bed. I had to take two to three naps a day. I literally couldn't stay awake," Carolyn said "If someone offered to pay me $1000 to stay awake for 15 minutes more, on some days, I just couldn't do it."

Then in the most insidious way, she began to experience problems with her vision. "I couldn't read signs that were far away like in the aisles at grocery stores." Because the problem occurred sporadically, she ignored it until the day she was driving alone to another city to pick up her children. "I started having trouble seeing and by the time I got to my destination, I couldn't see out of my right eye. It was all blurry and painful."

Carolyn was terrified. When she returned home late Friday afternoon, she saw an optometrist immediately, trying to get help before the weekend started. The optometrist told Carolyn that she had the worst dry eye syndrome she had ever diagnosed. The doctor told Carolyn that her corneas were so badly scarred that the light could not pass through them.

Although the doctor did not know what was causing her eyes to become that dry, it was critical to get moisture back into them in an effort to repair the corneas. Without delay, Carolyn began putting drops in her eyes. Later she worked with an ophthalmologist who used a prescription medication to help stimulate the moisture in her eyes. Although helpful, her condition never completely resolved, leaving her with some sensitivity and damage. She told the ophthalmologist that she was taking Prozac.

While trying to get her eye problem under control, new symptoms emerged. She began to lose her sense of smell and taste. With so many problems ravaging her body at one time, her doctor ordered an ANA blood test (anti-nuclear antibody test) which is used to help diagnose such autoimmune diseases as systemic lupus, scleroderma, Sjögren's syndrome, Raynaud's disease, rheumatoid arthritis, and autoimmune hepatitis. The test came back positive. She was diagnosed with Sjögren's syndrome which is a chronic disease in which white blood cells attack the moisture-producing glands. She was sent to a rheumatologist for steroid treatment. The doctor did a salivary gland biopsy, a painful procedure in which a small piece of salivary gland is removed for examination. It was thought that the biopsy would confirm Sjögren's syndrome but the results were negative.

"I was frightened and frustrated. The doctors could only offer me more tests which gave us no answers and more drugs which did not help me feel better. I was still extremely fatigued and feeling terrible," Carolyn said.

Then Carolyn brought her daughter to see me at The Block Center. While listening to my explanation of how I would approach her child's health problems, Carolyn had "an epiphany" as she described it. "I felt like Dr. Block would help me figure out what was really wrong with me instead of offering me more drugs. So I made an appointment to see her for me," she said.

As she had done with all the other doctors, Carolyn told me about all of her symptoms and that she was taking the drug Prozac. I picked up the Physician Desk Reference (PDR), a large book which reports the effects and side-effects of drugs. When I showed Carolyn the list of symptoms that Prozac can cause, all of her mysterious symptoms were there. Rather than coming off the drug "cold turkey," which can be dangerous, I helped Carolyn slowly stop using the Prozac. One of the dangers of dramatically stopping the medication is that the uncomfortable symptoms the sudden deprivation causes will make a dependent patient want to go back on the drug.

Once safely off the drug, Carolyn's debilitating symptoms stopped. Her energy level improved and her back and joint pain resolved. Within four weeks her vision returned. Once she was stable, I turned my attention to the underlying problem that had caused Carolyn to go on Prozac in the first place. She had felt tired and overwhelmed. She was a new mother of two children less than two years of age at the time she was first prescribed Prozac.

I suspected that Carolyn's problem was due to the extreme hormonal changes a woman goes through during and after pregnancy but most of her symptoms seemed to point to the thyroid. After running a comprehensive thyroid test, my suspicions were confirmed. Carolyn was hypothyroid, that is she had low thyroid levels which causes a slowing of the metabolism. This can lead to multiple symptoms including fatigue, depression, weight gain, insomnia, arthritis and rheumatic complaints, low sex drive, infertility, and skin problems.

Within three days of starting the thyroid replacement therapy, Carolyn was back to her old self. "I'll never forget. I think it was Thursday I started taking the thyroid medicine and when I woke up Sunday morning, I had a new lease on life. I felt wonderful," Carolyn said. "The fatigue lifted. I remember that Sunday was the first time I hadn't taken a nap in probably a year. I was productive and able to get so much done. I really felt great."

Carolyn recalled how during her final visit to the rheumatologist he had given her a prescription for sleeping pills saying that her fatigue was a result of not getting enough sleep at night. Carolyn had told him that she was sleeping all night as well as napping all day. Still he told her take the sleeping pills along with the Prozac and she would feel better.

"I want to speak out about what happened to me," Carolyn said. "I wouldn't want anyone to ever feel as bad as I did. I was not properly followed while on the drug and I didn't know the risks and dangers of quitting cold turkey. I wouldn't want any new mother to take a drug like Prozac during their pregnancy or while nursing when all they have is a hormone imbalance." Carolyn said that no doctor had performed a thyroid test on her during her pregnancies.

The number of adults who have been misdiagnosed with depression and are taking psychiatric drugs who come into my practice shocks me. Many women are being misled into thinking they have a psychiatric problem when it is actually a hormone imbalance that can be treated with natural, bio-identical hormones. Women should not be subjected to prescription antidepressants that come with the risk of serious side effects such as suicidal tendencies, heart problems and even death when their problem is actually hormonal.

Low thyroid levels and hormone imbalances are two of the most common causes of depressed feelings that are often overlooked. Only with a thorough history and a complete physical exam and lab tests can the true underlying medical causes of symptoms be diagnosed. Handing over a prescription after simply listening to the chief complaint is not sufficient. No patient should be treated that way yet I hear of experiences similar to Carolyn's every day in my practice.

Another woman had been taking Zoloft for 5 years. No thyroid test had ever been performed even though she had been pregnant and nursing while taking the Zoloft. If the test had been done, the doctor would have found what I did when I did a thorough thyroid evaluation. Every single thyroid marker was extremely abnormal. Her TSH (Thyroid Stimulating Hormone) was 76.2. Normal range is 0.4-5.5. I have never seen anyone with that high of TSH. Going through a pregnancy with a low thyroid condition like this placed her baby in extreme danger of mental retardation. And of course, the mother in danger of severe depression.

Being Depressed Is Not an Antidepressant Deficiency.

According to the FDA, an estimated 157 million prescriptions for newer antidepressants were dispensed to patients of all ages in the U.S. in 2002. (*Home News Tribune*, 8 March 2004) In that year an estimated 10.8 million prescriptions for the most widely used antidepressants were dispensed for patients under 18 years of age. (Mathews, A., 2004) Researchers at Washington State University found the rate of antidepressant prescriptions for children and adolescents more than tripled in the U.S. from the early 1990s to 2001. (Mathews)

From my own clinical experience I believe this can be attributed to a failure to order appropriate medical evaluations. The majority of my female patients who have been diagnosed with depression, post-partum depression, anxiety or PMDD (Premenstrual Dysphoric Disorder) and who have been prescribed psychiatric drugs do not have a psychiatric disorder. Normal life experiences or underlying medical problems actually lie at the heart of their symptoms.

Some Research Indicates SSRI'S May Increase Your Cancer Risk

Women taking antidepressants, especially SSRI's, may have a 7-fold increase in breast cancer risk. (Cotterchio, M., 2000)

One woman with whom I was talking was dying of cancer. She was taking an antidepressant. At the time of her diagnosis she had a one-year-old son. She had been fighting for her life for four years and she told me she had never shed a single tear. Thanks to the antidepressants she was not able to feel.

In a sense she could not grieve the loss of her own life or the loss of the opportunity to see her son grow. I believe at the same time the drug robbed her of this natural sadness it also deprived her of the strong emotional feelings she needed to fight her cancer.

When my mother was diagnosed with inoperable lung cancer and was given two months to live, I had her undergo a number of therapies along with radiation and chemotherapy. One component of her treatment was visualization, actively seeing herself fighting the cancer and driving it from her body. Had she taken antidepressants, I believe she would not have been able to wage an active war against her disease.

I also believe this ability to fight led to my mother's complete recovery. Four months after receiving a death sentence, she was pronounced free of cancer. She had no surgery. The disease, which originated in her lungs, had already spread. Her doctors believed that the treatment they offered to her would, at best, extend her life for a few more months.

No one believed that she would be cured. Now, seventeen years later, she has continued to be free of cancer. Then, had she been prescribed an antidepressant, I might not have known to stop her from taking it. I was a new doctor, out of medical training only six months. We cannot know if an antidepressant would have impeded her recovery but now, given my years of experience, I don't believe it would have helped.

Mental Illness, What Is It Anyway?

Mental: Pertaining to the mind
Illness: A condition marked by pronounced deviation from the
        normal, healthy state.
Mind: The psyche, the faculty or brain function, by which one is
        aware of his surroundings and by which one
        experiences feelings, emotions and desires, and is able
        to attend, reason and make decisions. (*Dorland's*
        Medical Dictionary, 23rd Edition)

Given the above definition "mental illness" would mean, " A

condition of the mind (psyche, faculty or brain function) marked by deviation from the normal healthy state." Who is deciding what a normal state is? There is no lab test or x-ray to prove a diagnosis of mental illness. I have a problem with the terminology and with the fact that people are being labeled with mental disorders in the absence of a proper medical work up.

Suffering people find a diagnosis and the prospect of a treatment for their problem comforting. They don't question the doctor, the diagnosis, or the resulting prescription. Without a complete physical exam and lab work a doctor simply cannot know what is wrong with an individual. When a new patient tells me they have been given a psychiatric diagnosis under these circumstances I cannot help but feel their previous doctor didn't know enough to find out what was wrong or was too lazy to try.

Invented Disorders

In his book, *The Myth of Mental Illness*, Psychiatrist, Dr. Thomas Szasz (2003) wrote:

> It is important to understand clearly that modern psychiatry — and the identification of new psychiatric diseases — began not by identifying such diseases by means of the established methods of pathology, but by creating a new criterion of what constitutes disease . . . whereas in modern medicine new diseases were discovered, in modern psychiatry they were invented. (p. 12)

By a show of hands, psychiatry votes on and establishes new rules to define "normal" and to diagnose "depression."

> According to the American Psychiatric Association, individuals who "have depression" must have their depressed symptoms for at least two weeks. The symptoms cannot be due to other physical conditions or illnesses nor can they occur as

the result of unexpected side effects of
medication or substance abuse. (APA, 2000,
p. 349)

No one has made clear what criteria led to the determination of
this short, two-week period. It seems to imply that the sadness
resulting from a death in the family or from some other life crisis
should pass in fourteen days. Given this expectation, anyone
who doesn't shape up in two weeks gets the psychiatric label
and the accompanying prescription for the antidepressant –
without having enough time to get an evaluation of the overall
physical condition (providing the diagnosing doctor even thinks
to order such a work up).

Psychiatry Is Subjective

Psychiatry has no objective basis to evaluate mental "disorders."
If a physical cause can be found for a psychiatric disorder, the
disorder ceases to exist. Since the American Psychiatric
Association (APA) states the symptoms cannot be due to other
physical conditions or illness, shouldn't that imply that the
diagnosing doctor actually evaluated the patient for these other
physical conditions or illness? I find this rarely occurs. I don't
think psychiatric labels should be used at all. At best they can
only be employed as a diagnosis of exclusion, when every other
possible medical condition has been evaluated and ruled out.
That rarely occurs. More often than not when the tests are
performed a physical cause can also be detected.

When you have a headache, you take an aspirin. If the headache
goes away, you don't worry any more about it. If it doesn't go
away, do you assume you have a mental illness? Of course not,
you try to find out why you are having a headache. Am I under
stress? Have I eaten today? Are my allergies acting up? Is it my
hormones? Is it high-blood pressure or a tumor? No one assumes
a headache is a mental illness. You go looking for the real cause
of the pain to fix it, not to mask it.

Autism Is Not a Psychiatric Disorder

When doctors don't know or don't take the time to find out what's wrong with a patient they often say, "It's all in your head," resorting to an informal version of the mental illness diagnosis that addresses only symptoms not causes. The manner in which physicians have dealt with autism offers a good example of this kind of flawed medicine.

Doctors originally couldn't find a reason for the symptoms exhibited by "autistic" children and so resorted to labels. At first the condition was considered a result of "Cold Mother Syndrome," shifting the blame for the child's problems onto poor parenting. Once such labels are applied they are hard to remove. Even though physical and medical problems have subsequently been found as possible causes of autism, for the past sixty years doctors have persisted in considering the condition to be psychiatric in nature.

I believe the initial application of the psychiatric label has actually kept the medical community from delving more deeply into the true medical causes for the symptoms autistic children present. Only in the last ten years has that begun to change as doctors like me are looking for and treating possible medical causes thus allowing children to see improvement or in some cases to recover from their symptoms. Conditions like heavy metal toxicity, nutritional deficiencies, auditory and visual processing problems, allergies and gastrointestinal problems can be possible causes. In the absence of the autism label, these advances might have occurred earlier and many more lives would have been saved from the consequences of the psychiatric diagnosis.

ADHD Is Not a Psychiatric Disorder Either

A similar reaction by the medical community has been applied to the attention and behavior issues that psychiatry has lumped into the label Attention Deficit Hyperactivity Disorder (ADHD). In evaluating children labeled and subsequently medicated for ADHD I have found real medical and educational reasons underlying their problems. When you treat the real cause you eliminate the need for the psychiatric label or for inappropriate medications. I have written extensively on this subject. For more information see my book, *No More ADHD*. (Block, M. A., 2001)

TeenScreen

In 2004, President George W. Bush signed a law that would provide funding for mental health screenings and drug recommendations based on a program designed in Texas by drug companies. The program, TeenScreen, already active in 43 states, uses incentives like free movie passes to encourage students to participate. (Richards, B., 2006)

Under this program schools have the right to use "passive consent." If your child does not return a form bearing your signature specifically forbidding the testing, it can be conducted without your permission. Lured by the promise of the reward, the child may never give you the form. Before you even know what is happening, your child could receive a psychiatric diagnosis and a drug recommendation.(Richards)

Mental Health Parity

Psychiatry has attempted to equate both mental and medical illness with mental and medical treatment. Some current laws require insurance companies to pay for mental and medical illness equally, which concerns me. High blood pressure, cancer and diabetes all have objective criteria. Mental illnesses do not. To require insurance companies to pay for something subjective could incur considerable costs. Any psychiatrist could say that anyone has a mental illness for any duration of time and no one could prove otherwise.

Who's Making the Money?

If a drug exists to mask symptoms of so-called mental illnesses, financial incentives exist to keep its use the status quo and to insure a market for its continued use. If medical causes for "mental" symptoms were found, the use of psychiatric drugs would be inappropriate. For that matter such findings would also invalidate the need for the psychiatrists themselves.

Both autism and ADHD, labeled as psychiatric disorders, have real medical and educational issues underlying the symptoms. The same is true of depression and calls into question the widespread use of antidepressant drugs to treat a psychiatric label rather than the true causes of a patient's suffering.

Fix It, Don't Label It

As a physician my job is to find the reasons for symptoms and if possible to fix them. Perhaps some people are content to have their symptoms only covered up with prescription drugs, but I think most would prefer to have the underlying cause accurately identified and remedied. At best psychiatric drugs only mask the problems, but there are cases in which the drugs can make the problems worse or cause new and potentially more serious issues.

Recently, I saw a young woman in my office who had been diagnosed with ADHD when she was younger and then later labeled as autistic. No lab work had been performed. She initially received a prescription for Ritalin and then an antidepressant for compulsive-like symptoms.

Ritalin, a substance akin to "speed," may have caused the compulsive symptoms but rather than discontinue the first drug and monitor her progress, the doctor added an antidepressant, which made the woman so groggy she could hardly stay awake during the day. Although a typical side effect of the antidepressant, the doctor administered a third drug for the extreme drowsiness. The three drugs he selected have never been tested together and each causes many of the same potential side effects including possible heart damage. Three drugs mean three times the risk.

No one listened to her heart. No one performed an EKG before the prescriptions were issued. No one evaluated and monitored her while she was taking the drugs. And no one ever looked to see what the true medical cause of her symptoms could be before exposing her to all those potential risks.

What's Your Doctor's Specialty?

As a patient, before you decide if a treatment is right for you, consider the specialty of your doctor. You can take the same symptom to five different specialists and come away with five differing opinions. Take a child with an ear infection to a pediatrician and you will probably get an antibiotic. An ear/nose/throat (ENT) doctor, who is a surgeon, might recommend surgery, placing tubes in the ear canal. An allergist might recommend an antihistamine and allergy testing.

A psychiatrist who sees an irritable child with problems focusing and who doesn't perform a physical exam to look for an ear infection might diagnose the child as ADHD. If I see the child and find the ear infection, I would recommend removing dairy products from the diet and instruct the parents in the performance of gentle, osteopathic manipulation to help drain middle ear fluids.

Even with the differing approaches to combat the problem, each of the doctors, me included, would have all done a physical exam. The psychiatrist usually does not. His diagnosis would be based on subjective symptoms alone.

"Psychiatrists Don't Do Physical Exams"

While I was a guest on *The Montel Williams Show*, another guest, a psychiatrist, told the American public plainly, "Psychiatrists don't do physical exams." Based on what my patients tell me, this would seem to be the common practice. Psychiatrists went to medical school. They are licensed physicians. Surely they learned to do a physical exam. It was a prerequisite for everyone in my medical school class. And yet psychiatrists routinely do not look for physical underlying causes for the symptoms with which they are presented. The only conclusion I can draw from this information is that psychiatrists must assume that if patients come to them they do so because they are mentally ill. The assumption guarantees the resulting diagnosis.

Not Just Psychiatrists

Unfortunately, psychiatrists aren't the only ones practicing this passive form of medicine. Far too many internists, gynecologists, pediatricians, neurologists and family practitioners simply listen to a set of symptoms and hand over a prescription. All too often the prescription is for a psychiatric drug.

No one would settle for this kind of care for his or her automobile. When we take a car to a mechanic we expect him to pop the hood and look at the engine. We don't put oil in the car without checking to see if the level is low. And yet we trust a psychiatrist who does not perform a thorough evaluation – no physical exam, no lab work – to hand us a drug, which we take with complete faith, most often in complete ignorance of its effects and potential side effects. Why would someone take better care of their car than they do of their body?

A Chemical Imbalance Is Not a Psychiatric Disorder

Psychiatry refers to many disorders as a "chemical imbalance." Both they and the pharmaceutical companies seem to imply that chemical imbalances validate the existence of psychiatric disorders. The chemicals to which they are referring, neurotransmitters, function in the body to communicate information nerve to nerve. Their levels normally fluctuate. We change the balance of our neurotransmitters every time we smile or frown. They are different when we are angry, frustrated, sad or happy.

If we do have too much of one neurotransmitter or too little of another, it does not mean we have a psychiatric disorder. These chemicals can become imbalanced as a result of thyroid or adrenal problems, hormone imbalances, nutritional deficiencies, allergies, low blood sugar, pain or any other medical problem or from a medicine side effect.

Feeling Sad or Depressed Is Not A Psychiatric Disorder

The reasons a person can become depressed are too numerous to list. Sometimes specific situations such as the loss of a loved one or some other tragic event triggers the depression. Some times people feel depressed because their bodies don't work properly. Depression is a normal response to death or loss, not a psychiatric disorder warranting medication.

The painful feelings represent the depth of our love for the person lost. To dampen those feelings does a disservice to the loved one and to the person who suffered the loss and needs to grieve. My grandmother died more than 30 years ago. She and I were close and her death was extremely painful to me. It still is. It took me a long time to stop crying every day. Even now as I write of her my eyes fill with tears. I don't cry because I am depressed but because I loved her and miss her dearly. My tears symbolize the strength of those feelings and the extent to which I treasure the time we had together.

Studies have found that crying can be healthy for us and not crying can be harmful. When I think of my grandmother now I don't feel depression but a mixture of pleasurable memories and painful loss, and with that the tears come. They are a more complex response than what the term "depression" can explain away. I would never want to lose those strong feelings and I would not want to take a pill that would not allow me to feel either love or loss.

Dr. Dear Abby

Everyone seems to be getting into the act of labeling people with psychiatric disorders. Even *Dear Abby* seems to push people to see psychiatrists and to take psychiatric drugs.

In one letter to *Dear Abby* that I recall reading, a young woman wrote that she was "tired all the time . . . I am overweight . . . completely burned out . . .. Maybe I should just lie down and die." In her reply, Jeanne Phillips said the young woman was exhibiting signs of depression and should seek treatment

(Phillips, J., July 5, 2003, p. 2F). This woman's symptoms could have been from low thyroid, adrenal fatigue, hormone imbalance, nutritional deficiency or even a brain tumor. Instead of zeroing in on depression as an easy answer, Phillips could have given her more sound advice: see a competent physician for a thorough evaluation to find out the real cause of the symptoms.

In another *Dear Abby* letter, a mother wrote that an uncle, a diagnosed schizophrenic, told her that her son had symptoms of mental illness. The mother wanted to tell the uncle to mind his own business. Phillips responded to the woman saying, ". . . mental illness can be genetic" and advised her to have her son evaluated (Phillips, J., Nov. 26, 2001, p. 4D). I believe she did the child a disservice by not suggesting a full medical exam but instead skipping straight to the psychiatric route.

The subjective nature of so-called psychiatric disorders also makes it impossible to objectively prove that they are genetic. Many of the medical problems that cause someone to feel depressed are genetic but it does not follow that mental illness is genetic.

In all fairness, however, Phillips' advice may be improving. I recently read a column in which she told a woman that it sounded as if she suffered from "postpartum depression," a condition caused from a hormone imbalance. Though Phillips still applied the label "postpartum depression" to a condition more accurately diagnosed directly as "hormone imbalance," she did at least link the two.

Depression Is Not Genetic

Often a patient tells me they are being treated for depression, that their mother had the same problem, or that depression "runs in the family." Somewhere along the way some doctor told them depression is genetic. It's more likely that the whole family suffered from "genetically" deficient medical treatment, the kind we've been discussing, that is characterized by insufficient evaluation and testing. As a result, generations of women lived and live with the belief that their genes predetermine their "mental" state.

The text of the *Diagnostic and Statistical Manual* supports this position by saying "a family history of depression would suggest a diagnosis of Major Depressive Disorder rather than a Mood Disorder Due to a General Medical Condition." (APA, 2000, p. 184) The tone of the phrasing in the DSM would indicate that the family history clinches the diagnosis, no need to look any farther or to consider possible medical factors.

When I think about family genetics as predicative of medical outcomes I remember one of my professors, Kim Korr. Both his father and grandfather died in their forties of heart disease and he expected the same fate. Instead of waiting to die, however, he began to exercise and to eat healthy and lived to be over 100.

Today, because of the human genomic project we have the capability to truly look at our genetic heritage. There are two things necessary for us to inherit and to manifest certain health problems, the genetic predisposition and an environmental insult. Certain genetic pre-dispositions are controllable. If we know we are predisposed, we can take steps to prevent the problems from occurring.

It would appear that people who experience drug side effects have a genetic predisposition for the problem in question whether they know it before taking the drug or not. Considering the role of genetic predisposition in the overall medical assessment lessens the randomness of the risk of such side effects. Simple blood tests can now help doctors predict which of their patients should not be given certain drugs. An understanding of a patient's genetic history *contributes* to a diagnosis but it does not *suffice* as a diagnosis on its own.

Find Information For Yourself

Before allowing a doctor to make assumptions based on the criteria in the DSM for diagnosing depression or falling victim to the assumption that depression (or any other condition) is genetic, educate yourself via the Internet and through the resources available at your local library. Have enough independent information and understanding to evaluate what your doctor is or isn't telling you.

Drug companies are successful because their products can deliver quick results, but being truly healthy takes a lot of work. Lifestyle changes may be in order. Many people don't want to be bothered with those kinds of changes. It's easier to take a pill and just feel better. Unfortunately quick fixes usually last only in the short term. Long-term resolutions mean receiving real medical evaluations and developing a commitment to making necessary and recommended changes.

The Medical Journals

In the journal, *Osteopathic Family Practice News*, (2002) Dr. Gregory James asserted that all adults should be "screened" for depression or anxiety during their periodic physical exams. He wrote that a nurse or medical assistant could do the screening. Such tell-tale signs as changes in hygiene, avoidance of eye contact, and responses to key questions were cited as potential indicators of depression. (James)

In fact, the article said that neither a physician nor a nurse was required to make the diagnosis. The patient himself could complete a questionnaire. The author referenced screening forms that could be used. These documents do not constitute a medical exam. They cannot be equated with lab tests or an MRI. They are only lists of symptoms to which the patient replies in the positive or negative. (James)

The article identified risk factors for depression present in various diseases, conditions, situations, environments and professions. The author contended that genetics play a role because certain personality types are more prone to depression. Other contributing factors could include cancer, chronic pain, weight loss or gain, disability, sexual dysfunction, gastrointestinal problems, heart diseases, vitamin deficiencies, hormonal imbalances, and alcohol or drug abuse. (James)

In addition the author identified certain drugs such as blood pressure and anti-Parkinson medications, tranquilizers and others as increasing the risk of depression. He then described what he believed to be common symptoms of depression: fatigue, headaches, pain, sexual dysfunction and gastrointestinal problems were included. The author first wrote that these were physical symptoms that place one at risk for being depressed then turned around and named them again as actual symptoms of depression. (James)

This circular reasoning presents a real problem. If the symptoms of a medical condition cause depression the physician would have to ignore that condition in opting to treat the depression with a psychiatric drug. That's simply bad medicine.

A nurse who works with the elderly population told me she felt there were not enough psychiatrists specializing in geriatrics. She went on to say that a man she knew began to have mental status changes. He was diagnosed with Dementia, a psychiatric diagnosis. The man was actually having a heart attack and was misdiagnosed with Dementia. This is why I am glad there are not more psychiatrists working with the elderly. The man needed a medical work-up, not a psychiatric label.

In "Understanding Depression in Women," Tanya Gregory (1999) wrote:

> Primary care physicians are becoming increasingly adept at identifying depression, although attributing a patient's symptoms to stress, anxiety or a physical illness when depression is the real cause is still a common mistake.

Gregory would seem to think finding and treating the actual physical problem to be a mistake. The article suggests that doctors not mention mental illness to their patient, but rather ask less confrontational questions first, "to show that you are actually listening to the patient and taking complaints seriously rather than leaping to the conclusion that she has no physical illness and the problem is all in her head." (Gregory)

Notice, she says to ask questions. She does not say to do a physical exam even though she implies earlier that there might be a physical illness causing the patient's symptoms. In fact, Gregory says that doctors are misdiagnosing by finding a physical illness and should diagnose depression instead. She appears to be telling doctors to pretend to be interested in their patients so the doctors will have more success in convincing the patient to take an antidepressant drug and that doctors should ignore physical signs and give their patients a diagnosis of depression.

This happened to my Mother when she saw a nurse practitioner in her doctor's office. When the nurse heard that my Dad had died recently, she immediately assumed my Mother was depressed. Though the nurse wanted to just prescribe an antidepressant, I insisted she do lab work on my Mother. My Mother had low potassium causing her symptoms. She did not have depression.

Gregory additionally suggests that if a woman does not wish to take a prescribed psychiatric drug such as an antidepressant, the doctor should try to convince her to take it by comparing the treatment to those for diabetes or hypertension. I have heard many doctors say, "If you had diabetes, you would take insulin, so taking an antidepressant for depression is the same thing." I strongly disagree. There is no valid comparison here. Diabetes and hypertension are real medical conditions that can be objectively diagnosed. Depression cannot. (Gregory)

In *Organic Psychiatry, The Psychological Consequences of Cerebral Disease*, (Third Edition, 1978), William Alwyn Lishman wrote, "The more one suspects an organic basis for the patient's mental condition, the more important will be the physical examination." Lishman goes on to cite a 1989 study (Koran, et al) in which a thorough evaluation revealed that almost 40% of patients in the California mental health system suffered from an important physical disease. "Relevant conditions included organic brain syndrome, epilepsy, migraine, head injury, diabetes and thyroid and parathyroid disorders." (Lishman, p.95)

According to Lishman the causes of the organic reactions range from degenerative, space-occupying lesions (tumors) to trauma, infections, vascular conditions, epilepsy, metabolic or endocrine imbalances, toxic substances, heavy metal toxicity, oxygen deprivation, or vitamin deficiencies. (Lishman, p. 153) Some patients with purely depressive symptoms were found "to respond to thyroxin (thyroid medication) . . . [when] . . . other forms of treatment . . . failed." (Lishman, p. 154). Lishman also states "The correct appraisal of patients with organic psychiatric disorders is a test of both psychiatric and general medical skills." He specifically cites the importance of a detailed differential diagnosis. (Lishman, p. 176).

A Differential Diagnosis

The basic and fundamental way my professors taught me to practice medicine involved specific steps: thorough history, complete physical exam, differential diagnosis, and informed consent. A differential diagnosis refers to all the possible problems that might cause a set of symptoms. Informed consent means that the doctor must tell the patient of all possible causes and treatments for the symptoms and of any possible side effects of the recommended treatments. If a doctor does not have the time or does not know how to rule out various conditions the patient should be referred to someone who can do those things. Above all, however, the temptation to rely on a simple psychiatric diagnosis must be rejected.

An acquaintance of mine who was initially diagnosed with a psychiatric disorder and medicated accordingly became steadily worse during his "treatment." Finally he received the work-up that should have been done initially. An MRI showed the presence of a brain tumor. It was removed and his symptoms resolved. Had his doctor provided a differential diagnosis, a brain tumor, among other possibilities, would have been explored. The tumor would have been found earlier and the prognosis would have been better.

Hypothyroidism Often Overlooked

I believe hypothyroidism to be one of the most commonly overlooked medical problems. Women (and even a few men) come to me with a prior diagnosis of depression. They report having taken antidepressants, feeling better for a short while, and then experiencing all the same symptoms again with greater intensity.

A good case to illustrate my point involved a patient who had seen various doctors over a thirty-year period, had been prescribed various antidepressants, but continued to suffer from the same symptoms. I performed a thyroid test and found the real cause of the symptoms – with one test – after thirty years. Some doctors will order tests, such as lab work for thyroid problems, and when the results are negative they assume the symptoms are "all in your head." I have found that the TSH, a single thyroid test does not constitute a thorough enough evaluation. (*See Chapter 4*)

In *Organic Psychiatry*, Lishman references many medical conditions that cause symptoms that look like psychiatric disorders. Unfortunately, having made those statements, the author follows a line of reasoning that contends that regardless of the medical conditions the symptoms are psychiatric. Never mind that once the physical condition is treated the psychiatric "disorder" goes away, which clearly indicates the problem was medical all along. (Lishman, pp. 595-745)

Referencing work done by Michael and Gibbons in "Interrelationships Between the Endocrine System and Neuropsychiatry," *International Review of Neurobiology*, (1963), Lishman lists potential underlying medical conditions including: hyperthyroidism, hypothyroidism, Cushing's, Addison's, diabetes, hypoglycemia, electrolyte disturbances, water depletion, sodium or potassium depletion, low calcium, low magnesium, low zinc, liver disorders, vitamin deficiencies, alcohol and drug (including prescription drugs) effects. (Lishman, pp. 5, 243-302, 514, 516, 519)

Conclusions

In the final analysis there is only one conclusion to draw. Just because you are depressed does not mean you have depression. Demand that your doctor perform the evaluations necessary to determine the true physical and medical conditions underlying your symptoms.

Chapter 2
The Diagnostic and Statistical Manual
or
Just Because It's Written Down, Doesn't Make It True

It is so easy to give a diagnosis of depression. All you have to do is ask the patient how they feel. The doctor does not have to do a physical exam or any lab work. Since there is no objective way to diagnose depression, the doctor can take the easy or lazy way out. As I have said before it is quick and cheap. But it has nothing to do with truly having depression. Depression is just a name and number in the *Diagnostic and Statistical Manual*.

The American Psychiatric Association writes and publishes the *Diagnostic and Statistical Manual* (DSM). This is a book that lists all the psychiatric diagnoses and the symptoms that define them. It also supplies code numbers that insurance companies use to identify the diagnoses. Doctors can use the codes and be paid by the insurance companies for doing nothing more than labeling the patient and writing a prescription. The DSM lists a Major Depressive Episode as a psychiatric disorder of:

> . . . at least two weeks [duration, characterized by] depressed mood or loss of interest or pleasure in nearly all activities. In children and adolescents, the mood may be irritable rather than sad. The individual must also experience at least four additional symptoms drawn from a list that includes changes in appetite or weight, sleep, and psychomotor activity; decreased energy; feelings of worthlessness or guilt; difficulty thinking, concentrating, or making decisions; or recurrent thoughts of death or

suicidal ideation, plans, or attempts. (APA, 2000, p. 349)

There is no explanation of who arrived at this definition or how and why two weeks constitutes a magic number. However a study published in *Psychotherapy and Psychosomatics* reports that 56% of DSM panel members (the individuals who write the DSM) had one or more financial associations with the pharmaceutical industry. One hundred percent of the panel members representing the 'Mood Disorders' and 'Schizophrenia and Other Psychotic Disorders' had financial associations with the drug companies. (Cosgrove, 2006) This appears to me to be a substantial financial conflict of interest.

The DSM goes on to say, "Some of the criterion items of a Major Depressive Episode are identical to the characteristic signs and symptoms of general medical conditions (e.g., weight loss with untreated diabetes, fatigue from cancer)." (APA, 2000, p. 351) Additionally the DSM contends that, ". . . a Major Depressive Episode is not due to . . . the direct physiological effects of a general medical condition (e.g., hypothyroidism)." (APA, 2000, p. 352). In other words, no one should be given a diagnosis of major Depressive Episode if they have a medical condition causing the symptoms.

From what we have learned so far, we know that psychiatrists usually do not perform physical exams or lab work. If they don't do such exams, they can't know if a patient has a medical condition. So, even though their own manual suggests that underlying conditions can cause the same symptoms as depression, it is much more likely that they will rule out a "general medical condition" in favor of a diagnosis of "Major Depressive Episode," which they will treat with antidepressant drugs because they have not performed a proper medical evaluation. And the panel members who make up the diagnoses have received money from the pharmaceutical companies whose drugs will be prescribed to treat those diagnoses.

Psychiatric Labels

In the absence of objective testing to determine the presence of mental illnesses the psychiatrists assemble every few years and talk about various groups of behaviors they think should be considered psychiatric disorders. They vote whether or not to include these disorders and their symptoms in the next edition of the DSM. By a simple majority, a new disorder is born and assumes a life of its own.

According to the Citizens Commission on Human Rights, a watchdog group that investigates and exposes psychiatric violations of human rights, within one year of the addition of ADHD into the DSM, some 500,000 children in the United States were diagnosed with the disorder. Today the number has climbed closer to 5 million. (Citizens Commission on Human Rights, 2005)

By its organizational structure and by the workings of the insurance industry, each new disorder receives a code number. The doctors use the code. The insurance companies pay the doctors. There's no mystery as to why the number of patients being diagnosed with a disorder grows after the disorder makes it into the DSM. The financial incentive to the doctors could not be more obvious. The diagnosis and treatment are fast and uncomplicated, freeing the physician to move on to the next patient, a much easier process than performing research and conducting tests. This flawed and subjective system has become the standard of care for psychiatric diagnosing.

The DSM Labels Real Medical Conditions as Psychiatric Disorders

The DSM codes used by doctors and insurance agencies to identify psychiatric disorders are not the only numbers in the book. The DSM also lists codes for general medical conditions that can cause the same symptoms as well as codes for medication-induced disorders. (APA, 2000, p. 409) The fact that both general medical conditions and those that are medication induced are present in the DSM amounts to a tacit admission on the part of the authors that the symptoms they identify as being psychiatric in nature can and do have other causes. In spite of this admission, time and time again a psychiatric diagnosis takes the place of a medical one.

For instance, the DSM does identify hypothyroidism, a medical condition that can be treated successfully, as a factor in depression. However the text clearly suggests that this physical problem should be classified as psychiatric, "Mood Disorder Due to Hypothyroidism." (APA, 2000, p. 405) Thyroid medication will make the depression go away. There is no need for an antidepressant or a psychiatric label. From my own clinical experience, I believe hypothyroidism to be the number one undiagnosed medical condition in adults causing depressed symptoms.

Hundreds of medical conditions affect how we feel. As long as doctors do not take into consideration these true medical conditions, more and more people will be labeled inappropriately and treated inappropriately. Not only will these patients continue to suffer from the same symptoms that led them to seek help in the first place, but they will also be exposed to new risks while taking the prescribed psychiatric drugs.

How the DSM Converts Medical Disorders to Psychiatric Labels

According to the DSM, "A mental disorder due to a general medical condition is characterized by the presence of mental symptoms that are judged to be the direct physiological consequence of a general medical condition." Additionally the text reads, "The purpose of distinguishing medical conditions from mental disorders is to encourage thoroughness in evaluation." The DSM uses the term "primary mental disorder" to indicate ". . . those mental disorders that are not due to a general medical condition . . .." (APA, 2000, p. 181)

The DSM recommends that a psychiatric diagnosis should be made when the history, physical examination, or laboratory findings indicate that the disturbance is not the direct physiological consequence of a general medical condition and not accounted for by another mental disorder. For instance, "... a family history of depression would suggest a diagnosis of Major Depressive Disorder rather than a Mood Disorder Due to a General Medical Condition." (APA, 2000, p. 184) This reasoning suggests that a physician may ignore a patient's medical condition if someone else in the family has been labeled with depression.

So even though the DSM continues to say that mental disorders are disorders that are not due to medical conditions, the written criteria in the DSM apparently captures every potential medical diagnosis and converts them into psychiatric ones. Any medical condition that makes the individual feel bad in any way automatically qualifies as a psychiatric disorder. Following this line of thinking, it would appear to me that the psychiatric profession actually believes life itself to be a psychiatric disorder.

You're Not Crazy. Your Doctor's Just Lazy.

On the subject of neurological and general medical conditions the DSM acknowledges that both "may cause personality changes." The text goes on to reference "physical examination findings, laboratory findings and patterns of prevalence and onset," which would imply that the psychiatrist or other doctor making the diagnosis actually does perform physical exams and lab work. (APA, 2000, p. 188-189) My experience indicates this rarely occurs.

Out of control blood sugar levels and hypothyroidism caused depression in one of my diabetic patients. According to the DSM, I should have diagnosed her with "Mood Disorder Due to Diabetes and Hypothyroidism." (APA, 2000, p. 404) Instead I referred her to an internist who adjusted her insulin and thyroid medication. Unfortunately, he also diagnosed her with depression and prescribed an antidepressant, a course of action that makes no sense to me.

Once her blood sugar and thyroid normalized so would her mood. The antidepressant only serves to dull all the feelings and in this case might prevent the woman from being fully alert to the symptom of low blood sugar or to the response of her other problems to medication. Symptoms are red flags that signal us when something is wrong. If the symptoms are covered up, the signals don't get through. Depression is a symptom, not a disease.

Chapter 3
Understanding the Medical System
or
If All You Have Is a Prescription Pad, Everyone Gets a Drug

People start out believing in the goodness of medicine. They have no reason to change that opinion unless they have misplaced their trust and been hurt as a result. This was certainly true for me. I believed in medicine. I believed that doctors were trained to help us get well and stay well. I believed that if a doctor gave me a prescription, I needed it.

Then a doctor gave me two prescriptions for my daughter. Michelle had chronic bladder infections when she was young. Though treated for years with antibiotics, her infections continued. Finally, her doctor prescribed psychiatric drugs – Valium, a tranquilizer and Tofranil, an antidepressant – for her bladder infections. I was not yet a doctor, only a mother who trusted her child's physician.

At the time I did question the use of such drugs. The doctor insisted Michelle would not get well any other way. I gave my child the medications. Michelle not only did not get well, she got worse. She had her worst bladder infection ever while taking Valium and Tofranil and became dependent on the drugs. When the doctor told me to stop the pills "cold turkey" Michelle went though obvious withdrawal. As a result and with the added complications of other side effects caused by the drugs, my daughter was sick for the next three years.

In my search to get my child well, I discovered what had really happened. The drugs prescribed to my daughter had never been tested for this use nor were they FDA approved for such use. Additionally the two medications had never been tested together and came with a host of potential and serious side effects. In self-defense and in defense of my child, I decided to go to medical school myself. I was determined to know what doctors know so that nothing like this would ever happen again to someone I loved. At age 39, I started medical school. I learned a great deal more than the practice of medicine.

The Pharmaceutical Companies Influence Doctors

Most patients and perhaps most doctors are unaware of the extent to which the pharmaceutical and insurance industries influence medical care. Without understanding these influences, you will not be able to make the best medical decisions for yourself.

Pharmaceutical companies strongly influence doctors from the first day of medical school. The PhDs who teach the basic science courses and the physicians who handle the clinical courses must obtain funding for their research. The pharmaceutical industry represents a large potential source for that funding. As a result, American medical educators fall under the sway of the pharmaceutical companies' agendas to the point that the relationship may actually constitute a financial conflict of interest.

Because medical educators were taught as they themselves are teaching, they don't even consider that there might be a better way. Many may not even realize the extent to which the pharmaceutical companies influence them and their teaching or they may try to deny the influence exists by justifying the money they receive as vital to their research. In truth the industry's power is so significant that many medical educators would not have jobs if pharmaceutical research money were unavailable.

Perks for Doctors

Practicing doctors must take a certain number of continuing medical education courses (CME). Physicians who present the course material are usually paid by pharmaceutical companies to give the lectures. Attendees accord respect to the speakers without always considering that they are, in essence, employees of the drug industry. Instead of coming away from the session with new and useful information, the "students" have learned exactly what the pharmaceutical company wants them to learn; prescribe our drug as the treatment of choice.

In a July 21, 2003 article for *The Wall Street Journal* journalist Gregory Zuckerman revealed that Biovail Corp., a large Canadian drug company, paid upwards to $1,000 each to thousands of U.S. doctors to prescribe the company's newly introduced heart medication. "The strategy, part of Biovail's effort to launch a medicine called Cardizem LA, underscores how some companies aggressively market their drugs to doctors." Taking their efforts a step further, Biovail paid as much as $150 to office managers to promote their product. Neither the physicians nor their office managers received "full payment unless they put 11 to 15 new patients on Cardizem LA." Zuckerman's research showed that some heart specialists found the Biovail drug to be no more effective than a cheaper, generic version of a similar medication. (Zuckerman, 2003)

When drug company representatives visit doctor's offices they come bearing lunch and other goodies for the staff. Although I don't prescribe enough drugs to warrant many visits from the drug reps, one did tell me that if a doctor were to prescribe a lot of their drug, the doctor could expect to receive a nice trip. The same rep confessed to me that going to see a doctor for a medical problem makes him uncomfortable because he knows that *he* actually trained the doctor.

Another pharmaceutical company representative told me that her company would hire doctors as "consultants" to encourage them to write prescriptions for their drugs. She was so uncomfortable with the ethics of her company that she quit and went into another field.

Pharmaceutical representatives are marketing products. It's business. Many doctors don't seem to realize this and think instead that these salesmen are educating them. The same companies host expensive dinners where their customers are "taught" by physicians on the corporate payroll. Some companies pay doctors for the use of their name as the "authors" of articles written for the sole purposes of publishing "research" beneficial to the sale of drug company products. The companies fill medical journals with full-page advertisements that help pay for the printing and mailing of the publications. It is not illogical to conjecture that those who are subsidizing the journal might influence the information printed in the journal.

The Drug Approval Process

Just because a drug has been tested and approved does not mean it is safe. The Food and Drug Administration (FDA) approves drugs for the market. Pharmaceutical company representatives and other individuals with direct financial conflicts of interest sit on FDA approval committees. I do not believe any drug can be considered safe as long as this system exists.

Take, for example, the approval of the Rotavirus vaccine. Though many dangerous side effects occurred in the testing of the vaccine, a majority of the committee members had a financial interest in getting it on the market. In spite of the known risks, the drug was approved and one year later was recalled because of the harm it caused. Children died from its use. Apparently the FDA ignored the dangers in favor of the financial gain that would flow to certain committee members. Use of the vaccine was discontinued but the flawed approval process stayed in place. I cannot help but wonder how many other dangerous, high-risk FDA approved drugs are still on the market for the same financially lucrative reasons. (Neergaard, 2002)

Journalist David Willman investigated controversy surrounding the diabetes drug Rezulin for *The Los Angeles Times*. He discovered that when an FDA medical officer questioned the drug's safety after reports that it caused liver damage, Dr. Richard C. Easan, the top diabetes researcher at the National Institutes of Health (NIH) and the supervisor for the drug's research as well as three other members of the study's executive committee said that they considered Rezulin's risk to be minimal. On their word, the FDA continued the study. Warner-Lambert, the manufacturer of Rezulin, collected $2.1 billion in sales before the drug was pulled from the market. It caused 556 deaths. Sixty-eight were from liver failure. (Willman, Dec. 7, 2003)

Easan, who repeatedly defended the drug, received more than $43,000 from Warner-Lambert for consulting services. When a participant in the NIH study died from liver failure, Easan and the other researchers withheld the information. At least 12 of the 22 researchers and the chairman of the study's data monitoring board (selected by the NIH to help conduct the nationwide study) received fees or research grants from Warner-Lambert. (Willman, Dec. 7, 2003, p. 10A)

According to the *AARP Bulletin*, (May 2006, p. 10), an FDA advisory board voted 8-1 to approve a new diabetes drug even though the risk of stroke and heart attack doubled in the clinical trials. The committee's chairman had performed work for the drug manufacturer. "The FDA has become too cozy with the industry it regulates . . . " said Senator Chuck Grassley, R-Iowa. (AARP) After Vioxx was pulled from the market, a panel voted to keep Celebrex and Bextra, two similar drugs, on the shelves. It was reported that nearly a third of the panel had ties to the drug manufacturers. "Had their votes been excluded, the drugs would not have gotten a positive vote." (AARP)

Problems With The Testing Process

Many drugs are approved after testing only a few hundred people for just a few months. After such drugs are released for sale, patients often receive prescriptions for years at a time with no testing to indicate potential side effects from long-term use. In August 2004 the *Los Angeles Times* exposed the content of a 20-page report that stated the NIH allowed more than 94% of its top-paid employees to keep their consulting incomes confidential. (Willman, Aug. 6, 2004)

The acceptance of drug company consulting fees by federal researchers at the NIH raises questions about the agency's ability to maintain independence in its scientific inquiries. The statement from the Office of Government Ethics quoted in the article described the NIH as beset with a "permissive culture" and called for firm, across-the-board restrictions to restore public confidence in the nation's preeminent medical-research agency. (Willman)

In part the *Los Angeles Times* article read:

> The head of the Office of Government Ethics, Marilyn L. Glynn, said in the report that without tougher standards, NIH "could give the appearance that some level of misuse of office is tolerable." The time had passed, she said, for trusting NIH leaders to make appropriate changes. The report is a setback for the director of NIH, Dr. Elias A. Zerhouni, who in June proposed banning agency directors and certain other top officials from taking industry payments while allowing most NIH scientists to continue to accept consulting deals. The acceptance of drug company consulting fees by federal researchers at the NIH has raised questions about the ability of the agency to maintain the independence in its scientific inquiries. (Willman, Aug. 7, 2004)

Dr. Curt D. Furberg, former head of clinical trials at the National Heart, Lung and Blood Institute, told Willman, "Private consulting fees tempt government scientists to pursue less-deserving research and to 'put a spin on their interpretation' of study results."

Are Drugs Safe?

The FDA does acknowledge that no approved drug should be considered safe until it has been on the market for at least ten years. Side effects that do not show up in a few months of testing may show up during long-term use. *The Journal of the American Medical Association* (JAMA) reported in its May 1, 2002 edition that "one in five new drugs [have] serious side effects that do not show up until well after the medicine has received government approval." (Temple, R., 2002)

The study, conducted at the Department of Medicine, Cambridge Hospital and Harvard Medical School concluded that:

> Recently approved drugs may be more likely to have unrecognized adverse drug reactions (ADRs) than established drugs, but no recent studies have examined how frequently post-marketing surveillance identifies important ADRs. (Temple)

More than ten percent of the 548 drugs analyzed that were approved by the FDA from 1975 through 1999 were later given a serious side-effect warning or were removed from the market.

> Adverse drug reactions are believed to be a leading cause of death in the United States. Prior to approval, drugs are studied in selected populations for limited periods, possibly contributing to an increased risk of ADRs after approval. Pharmaceutical companies frequently market new drugs heavily to both patients and clinicians before the full range of ADRs is ascertained. (Temple)

For years I have told my patients that taking new drugs amounts to playing Russian roulette. In an article for "The People's Pharmacy" a syndicated newspaper column, Joe and Teresa Graedon quoted Dr. Allen Roses, Vice President of Genetics at GlaxoSmith Kline, who said " . . . more than 90% of drugs work in only 30-50% of the people." The Graedon's compared the success of prescription drugs to buying a defective toaster. If the product doesn't work, we should ask for our money back. (Graedon, Jan. 19, 2004)

Researchers paid by the drug companies have a financial interest in the success of their research. I have seen medical clinics where patients appear to take a back seat to the research the doctor performs for a given drug company. Chances are good the doctor makes more money from the research than from the patients. I know a physician who has expressed vocal outrage at the effect of HMOs on his practice and income. He cannot make as much money since HMOs have taken over the practice of medicine. Now he conducts research for drug companies in his office.

Dr. John Mendelsohn, the president of M.D. Anderson Cancer Center in Houston, Texas, admitted that he has a financial interest in a drug that his center tested for the manufacturer, IMClone Systems. He also admitted that he should have informed his patients of this fact but he did not. As a board member and a major shareholder in IMClone, Mendelsohn clearly worked under a major financial conflict of interest. (*Washington Post*, June 30, 2002)

Pushing New Drugs Not Old

The pharmaceutical companies spend their time and money marketing new drugs, which they patent. According to "The People's Pharmacy" companies make $4 for each $1 they spend on advertising. (Graedon, Feb. 23, 2004) *Families USA* reports that pharmaceutical corporations actually spend almost twice as much on advertising as they do on research and development. *The Journal of the American Medical Association* indicates the companies spend between $8,000 and $13,000 per year on physicians in their efforts to get the doctors to prescribe their drugs. (JAMA, Jan 19, 2000)

A study published in the *New England Journal of Medicine* found the drug industry spent $15.7 billion for marketing in 2003. This would mean a profit of nearly $63 billion according to the ratio suggested by "The People's Pharmacy" article. This was an increase of 43% from 1997. A 1994 study in JAMA showed that doctors who asked for certain drugs to be added to the hospital list of approved drugs were more likely to have taken money from the drug manufacturers.

It would appear that the pharmaceutical companies do not encourage the prescribing of "old" drugs. Once a drug loses its patent, any other company can then produce it. These are called "generic" as opposed to "name brand" drugs. For example, "Prozac" is the brand name for a well-known antidepressant sold as the generic "fluoxetine hydrochloride," which is the medication's chemical compound. Generics are always cheaper.

One drug company representative told me that the only way I could get a sample of one of her older drugs was if I agreed to listen to her presentation and to accept samples of a new drug. I agreed because I have some patients who needed the old medication and could not afford it. I neither prescribed the new drug nor did I dispense the samples. When I read the product information about the new medication, I found that it caused cancer in mice during the FDA approval process and the rep could not answer any of my questions about this potential side effect. The newly patented drug went into the trash.

Do Anything to Keep a Patent

The manufacturer of Prozac, Eli Lilly, tried for six years to extend their drug's patent in order to keep generic versions from being produced. As journalist Rex W. Huppke explained in a 2001 article for the Associated Press, "That patent would have protected the Indianapolis-based company's monopoly until December 2003 and brought in an estimated $4 billion in sales for the company."

The Supreme Court rejected Lilly's appeal for the extension but the company began marketing a newly patented medication, Sarafem. According to their direct-to-consumer ads, Sarafem treats Premenstrual Dysphoric Disorder. (*See Chapter 5*) In reality, Sarafem is actually Prozac under a new name. There were many news reports exposing how the company renamed, re-patented and re-packaged the old drug. According to Lilly, the efficacy and safety of Sarafem was established in two studies. One was six months long and involved 320 patients. The other lasted three months and included 19 patients. (PDR, 2002, p. 1962) Remember Caroline in Chapter One? She had a bad reaction to

Prozac and her doctor prescribed Sarafem to her even after she told him she did not want to take Prozac. Fortunately she knew that Sarafem was just Prozac under a different name.

In recent years the drug companies have invested heavily in advertising directly to consumers, a profitable tactic, so profitable that $2.5 billion went into such campaigns in 2000. No one who has watched television, listened to the radio, read a newspaper or a magazine could miss the ads. Catch phrases like "ask your doctor if this drug is right for you" or "call now to find out how you can receive a free sample" have become so prevalent they are part of our television culture.

Are They Fooling You?

The pharmaceutical companies also use donations to non-profit groups to influence consumers. In February 2003 the *AARP Bulletin* exposed an organization called "Citizens for Better Medical Care." In one week the group spent more than $1 million in funds provided to them by the drug industry's trade association, The Pharmaceutical Research and Manufacturers of America (PHRMA). The money was used in efforts to influence elections. Not only do the drug companies get the benefit of the influence, they can also take a tax break for donating their money to the front groups.

The AARP also looked at a group called the "60 Plus Association" and determined it to be "a screen" for its efforts to defeat prescription drug legislation at the state level. These two groups and the "United Seniors Association" received millions of dollars in donations from the pharmaceutical industry. (Hogan, 2003)

I have suspected this sort of thing for years. I work extensively with children who have been labeled "ADHD" and given amphetamines as treatment. A non-profit group called CHADD, "Children and Adults with ADD," promotes the use of these drugs in children and consequently has received the same lucrative "donations" from the pharmaceutical companies that make the medications. Not only does CHADD encourage the use of these drugs, but in congressional testimony the group was also characterized as a conduit or channel of the drug companies, a pipeline for spreading their message directly to the public.

In 1995 the U.S. Department of Justice Drug Enforcement Agency (DEA) described CHADD and its activities in its Drug and Chemical Evaluation Section:

> CHADD, non-profit organization, which promotes the use of Ritalin, also receives a great deal of money from the drug manufacturer of Ritalin. CHADD does not inform its members of the abuse problems of Ritalin. CHADD portrays the drug as a benign, mild stimulant that is not associated with abuse or serious side effects. Statements by CHADD are inconsistent with scientific literature. In addition, The International Narcotics Control Board expressed concern that CHADD is actively lobbying for the use of Ritalin in children. (U.S. Department of Justice Drug Enforcement Agency Drug and Chemical Evaluation section,1995)

Pharmaceutical companies are in business to make money. They are good at it. The fact that these manufacturers do make important and effective drugs woos the public into thinking that everything they do is vital to the public's interest. I don't believe this to be true. As companies traded on the New York Stock Exchange, the pharmaceutical manufacturers do what benefits their shareholders.

The drug companies invest money to influence political campaigns with good results. When the National Home Security Bill was passed, former Texas Congressman Dick Armey (R) tagged on a benefit to the drug companies that would prevent anyone from suing such a company for side effects from a vaccine. He did it at the last minute and did not inform anyone that it had been added. When many were furious about the addition, he did not come forward and admit that he was responsible for the rider for many days. (CBS Evening News, December 12, 2002)

Government Betrayal

Protecting patients in the face of drug testing problems, inadequate FDA approval methods, and the enormous influence of the pharmaceutical industry grows harder each day. *The New York Times* reported that the Bush administration has been going to court to block lawsuits by consumers who say they have been injured by prescription drugs and medical devices. The administration contends that consumers cannot recover damages for such injuries if the Food and Drug Administration has approved the products. Patients and their families involved in these lawsuits described a sense of having been betrayed by their government. (Pear, 2004.)

Great Britain Bans SSRIs in Children

Recently, Great Britain banned the use of SSRI (Selective Serotonin Re-uptake Inhibitors) such as Prozac, Paxil and Zoloft in children and teenagers. The ban was based on information regarding an increased risk of suicide in these populations. In a trial of Paxil, children were found to be nearly three times more likely to commit suicide while taking the medication. (British Medical College of Psychiatry, Feb. 19, 2005)

Officials in Great Britain issued a statement that said in part, "It has become clear that the benefits in children for the treatment of depressive illness do not outweigh these risks." Nine days later in the United States the FDA issued a similar warning. A member of the British Parliament, Paul Flynn, blasted the use of Seroxat (the European name for Paxil):

> I believe that need for the drug is based on a great myth: the idea that we can go through our entire life in a state of continuous euphoria and that if we suffer a moment of discomfort, pain, boredom, grief or anxiety

we should be classified as ill and in need of
medicine. . . . [this] scandal is one of
gigantic proportions that affect millions of
people. (Flynn, 2004)

The trust of the patients was abused when doctors administered
a medication, Paxil, that turned mild stress into suicidal despair
and a passing anxiety into a lifelong addiction. (Flynn)

Clinical trials of Paxil, Zoloft and Effexor found their
effectiveness to be no better than a placebo. Sixty-nine percent of
those taking Prozac indicated they continued to have depressed
feelings. Fifty-nine percent of children studied responded just as
well to a "sugar pill." During the first four years Prozac was on
the market 350 people taking it committed suicide. (Waters,
2004)

On March 23, 2004, the FDA asked makers of 10 antidepressants
to add or to strengthen suicide-related warning on their labels.
In its statement the FDA stressed that people prescribed
antidepressants need to be closely monitored for signs of suicide
including agitation, anxiety, irritability, and recklessness. In the
presence of any of these symptoms doctors should consider
lowering the dosage or slowly discontinuing use of the
medication. (FDA Public Health Advisory, 2003)

In February 2004, families that suffered adverse affects of mind-
altering drugs known as SSRIs testified at a hearing of the Food
and Drug Administration. Glenn McIntosh, a father who
testified, described how his 12-year-old daughter Caitlin
Elizabeth McIntosh committed suicide just eight weeks after
being put on Paxil and then Zoloft. She suffered from a mild
seizure disorder. The drugs were intended to help her sleep and
to cope with the onset of puberty. (O'Meara, 2004)

When Caitlin did not do well on Paxil, the family physician took
her off the medication "cold turkey," a dangerous and
inappropriate action. A week later the child saw a psychiatrist
who put her on Zoloft. It was then that Caitlin began to
experience strong suicidal ideations, along with severe agitation

known as akathisia, and hallucinations. Next she was admitted to the adolescent ward of a mental hospital to "balance her meds." (O'Meara)

The story, in her father's words, is even more tragic and compelling:

> . . . there, things only got worse, as she was put on other strong psychotropic drugs to treat the symptoms that we now know were actually caused by the SSRIs. And let me be very, very clear about something: The dramatic and severe symptoms that led to my daughter's suicide manifested only after she started taking antidepressant drugs.
>
> The downward spiral continued until Jan. 5, 2000, when she hung herself with her shoelaces in the girl's bathroom in the middle school she was attending. We were told that antidepressants like Paxil and Zoloft were wonder drugs, that they were safe and effective for children. We were lied to. The pharmaceutical companies have known for years that these drugs could cause suicide in some patients. Why didn't we? I implore you, ban the use of antidepressants here in the United States so that other parents will not have to endure the pain I've felt and other children might be saved. (O'Meara)

In spite of these incidents the number of prescriptions written for antidepressants continues to rise. The FDA estimates that sales of antidepressant drugs in the United States increased from 14 million in 1992 to a staggering 157 million in 2002. (*Home News Tribune*, 2004) Far too many of those prescriptions are for children, about 11 million in 2002. Of those, 2.7 million were for children 11 and under. (Barrett, 2004) Mark Olfson, a professor of clinical psychiatry at Columbia University, estimated approximately 1 percent of children in the United States are treated for depression each year, with 57 percent of those receiving antidepressants. (Vedantam, January 29, 2004)

When questioned by the FDA, drug company representatives explained the suicides by saying that the depression that necessitated the use of their drugs in the first place caused the patients to take their own lives. (Patterson, 2004) Don Farber, a harsh critic of Paxil manufacturer, Glaxo-SmithKline (GSK), said that GSK manipulated the data on Paxil-related suicides. GSK claims Paxil actually decreased the number of suicides while suicides in those taking a placebo increased. Farber, however, contends that only one placebo patient out of 554 committed suicide compared to the 49 out of 2,963 on Paxil. (Patterson) If he is correct, nine times more people committed suicide while taking Paxil.

On January 29, 2004 *The Washington Post* revealed that the manufacturers of SSRIs might be withholding important safety information from the public.

> Makers of popular antidepressants such as Paxil, Zoloft and Effexor have refused to disclose the details of most clinical trials involving depressed children, denying doctors and parents crucial evidence as they weigh fresh fears that such medicines may cause some children to become suicidal. (Vedantam, Jan. 9, 2004, p. A01)

According to the article, the companies say that the studies are trade secrets. Researchers familiar with the unpublished data said the majority of undisclosed trials show that children taking the medicines did not get any better than children taking dummy pills. (Vedantam)

Although the drug industry's practice of suppressing unfavorable data is legal, doctors and advocates say such secrecy distorts the scientific record. Vera Hassner Sharav, a critic of the drugs and a patients' rights advocate told Vedantam, "Conflicts

of interest and the company control of the data have thrown out the scientific method. If hundreds of trials don't work out, they don't publish them, they don't talk about them."
Philip Perera, a medical director at GlaxoSmithKline, said he preferred to publish the results of all trials but that negative studies could lead doctors to prematurely reject a medicine. "If you start publishing negative data, will it be concluded by practitioners and others that the drug is ineffective?" he asked, saying that genuinely effective medicines sometimes do no better than placebos, or dummy pills, in trials. (Vedantam)

Following that line of reasoning we should also say that positive studies must lead doctors to prematurely accept a medicine, which I believe the pharmaceuticals companies would prefer. A completely unbiased study might well show that a significant number of people get better without any medication. The results of trials conducted under the auspices of the drug companies will be limited to a conclusion on the profitable use of the drugs not on the real outcome of the research.

In three trials of Paxil conducted by GlaxoSmithKline on depressed children the bias towards drugs was evident. All three studies showed that children on the drug did not do better than those on placebos but the company released the results of only one trial. Based on this data, the company warned British doctors that Seroxat (the European name for Paxil), "should not be prescribed as new therapy" in depressed children younger than 18, citing a risk of increased hostility, agitation, and suicidal thoughts and attempts. No such warning was issued in the United States where the company's public statement regarding the use of Paxil for children was, "No recommendations can be made regarding the use of Paxil or PaxilCR in these patients." (Vedantam)

Dr. Lawrence Diller, a Walnut Creek, Calif., pediatrician and author of "Should I Medicate My Child?" told *The Washington Post*, "As a front-line doctor dependent on research, it seems so contaminated by potential conflicts of interest . . .. The smoking gun is revelations from the British that negative studies were not published." (Vedantam)

Many scientists advocate clinical trials paid for with public dollars to ensure the purity of the science. As a result, the National Institute of Health has expanded its funding of such studies. "We have been dependent on the pharmaceutical industry to provide the answers," said Thomas R. Insel, director of the NIH. "The questions they want answered are different than the public health questions." (Vedantam)

FDA Involved in Cover Up

In another *Washington Post* article by Shankar Vedantam, it was revealed that top FDA officials told an FDA medical officer to delete information on antidepressant risks from records submitted to Congress. According to a bipartisan Congressional panel, the FDA prevented Andrew Mosholder from presenting conclusions that antidepressants increase suicidal thoughts and behavior in children. As long ago as 1996, an FDA official suggested that there may be an increase in suicide in children taking Zoloft but there did not appear to be any follow-up. FDA officials said they did not wish to frighten parents from using the drugs. (Vedantam, Sept. 24, 2004)

A doctor may prescribe an FDA approved drug for anyone for anything regardless of whether or not the substance has been tested for that use or with that patient population. With this "off label" use, unexpected results and side effects can and do occur. I have never understood why doctors are willing to take that risk.

The rise in off-label prescriptions being handed out each year proved alarmingly high when Knight-Ridder journalists Alison Young and Chris Adams conducted a six-month investigation of the practice in 2003. Over a five-year period the number of such prescriptions rose to 115 million annually in spite of the resulting injuries and deaths.

This is an issue of concern dating back to 1962 when thousands of Americans had been deformed by thalidomide. The United States Congress ordered the Food and Drug Administration to take steps to prevent such a thing from ever happening again. It was during this remaking of our nation's drug safety regulations that lawmakers began to worry pharmaceutical companies might get medications approved for one use but promote them for others. The FDA subsequently reviewed the 3,443 drugs then on the market and deemed one-third to be useless. (Young & Adams)

The agency has the power to require drug companies to prove the safety and effectiveness of off-label use but in a 1996 deposition Dr. Robert Temple, speaking for the FDA, said, "We think about this [requiring such proof] all the time . . . We just don't know quite how to do it." (Young & Adams)

As difficult as it may be to comprehend, attempts to strengthen the regulatory power of the FDA on the matter of off-label drug promotion boils down to an issue of free speech and the often-slippery definition of commercial speech. What should be an issue of medical safety has instead become one of Constitutional semantics. (Young & Adams)

Nothing illustrates the ineffectiveness of the FDA more clearly than the re-introduction of thalidomide into the U.S. market. In 1998 the drug was approved to treat a leprosy-related skin condition virtually unheard of in this country. But Celgene Corp. has aggressively promoted thalidomide for treating multiple myeloma, a form of cancer. As of 2003 seventy percent of thalidomide prescriptions were written for myeloma with only one percent going for the approved use. (Young & Adams)

Instead of clamping down on the practice of off-label prescriptions, the FDA has actually considered granting the drug companies greater latitude to promote such untested therapies. (Young & Adams) Claiming that recent court rulings have eroded the agency's power, FDA officials have sought public comment on whether drug makers should have more freedom to market unapproved uses for their drugs. In reality, the FDA suffers from conflicted mandates: get powerful drugs to market, protect the public, respect the First Amendment, regulate drug company advertising, allow doctors the freedom to practice, but prevent doctors from making mistakes with prescriptions. The situation allows for a myriad of exploitable loopholes and for terrible misuses of off-label medications. (Young & Adams)

Young and Adams found doctors prescribing the asthma drug Terbutaline for premature labor, epilepsy drugs like Topamax being used as antidepressants, and the anti-psychotic Risperdal administered for anxiety. Although technically legal and even defended by the American Medical Association, off-label prescriptions have been responsible for heart attacks, nerve damage, strokes, and blindness. (Young & Adams)

Tammie Snyder, a Michigan woman who received Terbutaline via a pump attached to her thigh for three and a half months at the end of her pregnancy delivered two healthy baby girls but within days suffered heart complications so severe a transplant was considered. She was later told that future pregnancies would be too hard on her heart. (Young & Adams)

Topamax, approved by the FDA in 1996 as a supplemental epilepsy treatment, causes numbness and tingling in the hands and feet, depression, kidney stones, impaired memory, and vision problems that can result in blindness. The drug has become a popular off-label treatment for migraine headaches, schizophrenia, bipolar disorder, depression, pain, nerve damage, and obesity. Carolyn Bartley, 44, of Annapolis, MD took Topamax for one week for bipolar disorder and required laser surgery in both eyes to restore her vision. "Everywhere I looked, it was like a watercolor painting, and somebody had smeared it," she said. (Young & Adams)

An 85-year-old Texas man, suffered a series of stroke-like attacks after receiving Risperdal for "cancer phobia." Used as an off-label treatment for Alzeheimer's and dementia, more than 670,000 Risperdal prescriptions were written in 2001 generating $929 million in retail sales. Johnson & Johnson, the maker of Risperdal had been privately aware of issues with the medication for two years before admitting the fact and issuing a warning about its use for elderly patients. (Young & Adams)

Most doctors do not see enough patients in their practice to accurately assess the success or failure of the off-label treatments they favor. Such prescriptions may continue for years before clinical trials are conducted that reveal the use to be either harmful or useless. In far too many cases such trials are never conducted. (Young & Adams)

Making drug samples freely available to doctors further encourages off-label prescriptions. Of particular concern is the practice of giving specialty drugs to non-specialist physicians. This promotes the benefits of a given drug on slim evidence at best and can lead to tragedies. When Memphis, Tenn. Cardiologist Dr. Gary Murray could not arrive at a diagnosis for his 71-year-old patient's chest pains after a battery of tests, he gave Milton Cole a prescription to help blunt the pain and some free samples of Prozac. (Young & Adams)

Murray was unaware of the debate raging among experts that Prozac could induce suicidal tendencies. Thirteen days later Cole's wife found him hanging from a beam in the back room of their shop. "This was a patient of mine, and I was trying to help him. I'm completely upset . . . I'll be that way forever," said Murray. "I chose Prozac probably because I had samples of it. I thought it was a pretty harmless thing to do." (Young & Adams)

Drug companies have every reason to continue to foster a symbiotic relationship with physicians. Off-label sales of top-selling drugs totaled $12.9 billion in 2002. That same year the value of samples given to physicians reached $11.9 billion, drugs dispensed by an army of 94,000 drug company sales representatives – one rep for every seven doctors in the United States. (Young & Adams)

In reality federal law prohibits drug makers from advertising off-label drug use and since 1998 the FDA has cited companies seventy times for violations of this restriction. That does not mean, however, that off-label promotions are not commonplace. Cephalon, Inc., based near Philadelphia, relies so heavily on off-label sales that a Wall Street analyst cited the practice as a reason to invest in the company. "From 2000 to 2003, 60 percent of Cephalon's sales were of Gabitril or Provigil, two drugs for which the majority of the written prescriptions are off-label."

Provigil, a medication approved for narcolepsy (pronounced sleepiness) has been prescribed for multiple sclerosis fatigue, ADD, depression and "miscellaneous fatigue." Gabitril, an anti-seizure drug, was given off-label for pain. (Young & Adams)

In a 1998 court brief lawyers for the FDA said:

> While physicians may believe that they are
> in a better position than [the] FDA to
> evaluate off-label claims, both the evidence
> and the law say otherwise . . . Physicians
> tend to have confidence in their own ability
> to critically assess off-label information. The
> studies demonstrate, however, that such
> confidence is often unwarranted and
> incorrect. (Young & Adams)

If your doctor has given you an off-label prescription ask why and press the point. Find out if your doctor has researched the use of the drug in the suggested manner and on what he bases his conclusions. Ask about alternate treatments. Find out about the side effects. Don't just trust what you're told. Do the research yourself. Don't depend on the leaflet that comes with the medication. Talk to your pharmacist or look up the drug on the Internet. (Young & Adams)

Drugs vs. Cure

I do not believe that pharmaceutical companies make any attempt to cure diseases. Cures mean no need for more drugs and no more profits. High blood pressure medications serve as a good example of this situation. I was taught that we do not know the cause of 90% of high blood pressure cases. The drug industry produces many drugs to lower blood pressure but I am not aware of any research to find the actual cause for the 90% of unexplained cases. Personally, I have found several reasons for high blood pressure in my patients. Allergies and nutritional deficiencies are two of these causes. When I treat what I find, the blood pressure normalizes and no blood pressure medicine is needed. However, this approach does not sell drugs.

Insurance-Do You Know What You're Paying For?

Although more subtle than the effect of the pharmaceutical industry, insurance companies have a profound effect on your medical care. When you pay your premium the insurance company essentially bets you will not have more medical bills than what you have paid them to cover. People seem to think that the insurance company should cover all their health expenses. However, the cost of insurance will just keep increasing with that kind of thinking. The insurance company is always going to make a profit, so your premiums will always go up to cover any increases in your medical expenses.

You get what you pay for. If your insurance plan is less expensive, you will have fewer services covered. With the HMO system, the individual subscriber receives fewer options than the person who has indemnity insurance. With the HMO, you will have to choose from a set of specific doctors and be satisfied with a set of specific services. With an indemnity policy, you can go to any doctor you choose and have a specific amount paid for their services.

I am a believer in the old type of insurance. This would make each family accountable for their doctor's office expenses but have an insurance policy to cover additional bills that may occur. This used to be called "hospitalization insurance" because it was used when someone had a large expense like being in the hospital. Today it would be called a Health Savings Account. This system cultivates more patient responsibility. If you are paying out of your own pocket, you will not overuse your doctor's services. Today, with the HMO model, people with problems that they know are not very serious and will heal on their own may tend to go to the doctor just because the HMO will pay for the visit. I have observed that since the HMO system came into being, doctors do not spend as much time with patients. If the doctor can get the patient in and out quickly, they can see a lot more patients and get a lot more co-payments. I believe this is why the antidepressants have been used so much. If the doctor does not have to spend time with the patient or spend money on lab work or other medical services, but rather make a diagnosis from a brief interview and hand over an antidepressant prescription, they can move on to the next person.

Today many insurance programs dictate certain guidelines in your treatment that your doctor must follow. The insurance company tells your doctor which drugs may be prescribed, a policy that may not have anything to do with the best treatment for the problem. The guidelines usually stipulate the use of the least expensive treatment first. When the HMO programs first began in Texas I attended a meeting to learn more about them. The speaker suggested that if an older person came in needing a hip replacement, the surgery should be delayed in favor of giving the patient a walker and hoping they died before the operation was required. I stood up and walked out. I have no intention of practicing that kind of medicine.

Many people are surprised to find that I do not accept medical insurance but run my office on a "fee for service" basis. The patient pays for the services they receive at the time they receive them. I give them a bill that can be used to file with their insurance company. If my office handled the filing I would have to hire more staff to do nothing but spend their time going after reimbursement for my services from the patient's insurance company. This makes no sense to me.

You, the patient chose the insurance company. You chose it for its cost or for what it offers. The doctor should not be expected to deal with the insurance company that you chose. Some of my patients have remarked that after dealing with their own insurance company, they now understand why I don't accept their insurance policy for payment. Some have spent weeks or months trying to get reimbursed. If a doctor has to do that, they cannot be free to provide the medical care you deserve. Your relationship with your insurance company is your choice and your business. I don't belong in the equation.

The insurance companies have a great deal of influence over what happens to you as a patient. They decide which services will be covered and which will not. The individual at the other end of the phone line making the decision on your medical care may not have any medical background. They may have been told to deny your claim automatically. The insurance company may be counting on their clients not fighting rejected claims thus upping the corporate profit margin. But I have observed that when such objections are raised the company will often make the payment in the end.

In 2001 the Kaiser Family Foundation released a report pointing to widely disparate approaches by insurance companies in regard to depression. As part of the study, the health research group created several hypothetical applicants and sent them out to get insurance. While insurers responded consistently with most of the "applicants," there was no agreement on what to do with "Emily," a healthy 56-year-old woman who started taking a low dose of Prozac following her husband's death the previous year. Twenty-three percent of the insurers surveyed rejected her, another 23 percent quoted her a higher rate, 12 percent offered her benefits that excluded treatment for mental disorders and 27 percent offered her both higher rates and limited benefits. (Sanders, 2004)

Another Drug Pusher

The insurance companies along with the pharmaceutical companies appear to me to encourage drug-based medicine. Giving out a quick diagnosis and a prescription does not tie up the doctor's time so more patients can be seen in a day. The less lab work ordered and fewer tests performed the more money the insurance companies save.

No one can safely assume that the prescription they receive represents the best treatment for their problem. More likely it reflects the limitations of any particular doctor or the latest product of a given pharmaceutical company or the restrictions placed by the insurance company. If the only tool that doctor has is a prescription pad, then everyone is going to get a prescription. If the doctor has recently attended a meeting sponsored by a drug company or has been visited by a drug company representative, those encounters will likely affect the writing of the prescription. Until the public questions the role of such practices and influences in our health care system, they will continue unchecked.

Now let's look at the real causes of the symptom called depression.

Section II

Find the Cause — Fix the Problem

What They Don't Want You To Know

Chapter 4
The Thyroid and Adrenal Glands
or
If They're Not Working, You're Not Working

After seeing an endocrinologist for seven years, Kevin, a young man in his thirties, described symptoms to me that sounded like hypothyroid. The endocrinologist had tested him for hypothyroidism but with negative results. Kevin, however, was only tested for TSH levels. When I re-tested him with a more complete screening, Kevin did have hypothyroidism. Upon reviewing my test results, the endocrinologist prescribed thyroid medication. I wonder why the endocrinologist had only tested TSH for seven years and also if the experience will affect the thoroughness of the doctor's future testing procedures.

The thyroid is often mentioned as an underlying cause of many symptoms labeled as mental illness. In spite of this, I see many adults and children who have been given diagnoses of depression, Pre-Menstrual Dysphoric Disorder (PMDD), autism or Attention Deficit Hyperactivity Disorder (ADHD), but have never had a simple thyroid test.

I saw one young boy diagnosed with serious depression who had been prescribed a Selective Serotonin Re-uptake Inhibitor. (Drugs in this category include Prozac, Paxil, Zoloft, and Luvox, Effexor and others.) His prescription had not been tested on young children and was not indicated for use in that population. The drug did not relieve his symptoms. He had not received a thorough physical exam or a series of lab tests, especially a thyroid test. I performed the test and found him to be hypothyroid. With thyroid replacement treatment the child felt much better and his parents and teachers said he was like a different person. He did not need the antidepressant. Just because he was depressed didn't mean he had depression.

Another young boy in my practice had been diagnosed as ADHD and received Ritalin. The drug not only did not improve his condition but also caused him to have seizures. He too proved to be hypothyroid. Unfortunately, when the Ritalin was stopped the seizures continued. Side-effects do not always resolve when the drug is discontinued. I see many cases like these each year, often with the psychiatric diagnosis of ADHD or depression, but never with a history of complete thyroid testing.

Understanding the Thyroid

Dubbed the "the master gland" for its control of all metabolic processes in the body, the thyroid regulates temperature, brain function, circulation, and nerve and muscle health. Located in the front of the neck just below the larynx, the thyroid gland secretes the hormones thyroxine (T4) and triiodothyronine (T3). When this gland malfunctions – most commonly as hypothyroidism or hyperthyroidism – the resulting imbalances can cause symptoms of depression.

The thyroid gland functions to take the iodine found in many foods and convert it into T4. T4 then must convert to T3 which is actually the active form of thyroid. The lab measurement for T3 is "free T3", something I find is rarely measured. When the level of T4 drops too low the pituitary gland produces Thyroid Stimulating Hormone (TSH) to increase the T4 secretions. The level of TSH in turn drops as the T4 levels increase. When this process breaks down in some way thyroid "problems" result. (Two good books on the subject are Broda Barnes and Lawrence Galton, *Hypothyroidism, The Unsuspected Illness* and David Brownstein, *Overcoming Thyroid Disorders*.)

Hypothyroidism

Hypothyroidism, or under activity of the thyroid gland, causes a variety of symptoms as it slows the body's normal rate of function. These may include:

- depression
- fatigue
- weakness

- cold intolerance
- constipation
- weight gain (unintentional)
- joint or muscle pain
- thin and brittle fingernails
- dry, thin and brittle hair
- pale color
- dry and flaky skin
- puffy hands and feet
- decreased taste and smell
- abnormal menstrual periods

Hyperthyroidism

Hyperthyroidism, or thyroid gland over activity, may occur naturally or as a result of taking thyroid medication. In the latter case it is extremely important to monitor the individual's thyroid levels until their medication is properly regulated. Too much thyroid can cause:

- end of day fatigue but difficulty sleeping
- trembling hands
- hard or irregular heartbeat (palpitations)
- increased blood pressure
- shortness of breath
- chest pain
- muscle weakness
- irritability, easily upset
- increased risk of osteoporosis
- weight loss
- diarrhea
- abdominal cramps
- sweating
- heat intolerance
- menstrual irregularities

Older people with hyperthyroidism may just lose weight or become depressed.

Issues With "Standard" Thyroid Testing

How to best test for thyroid problems continues to be debated. In general, doctors measure the TSH blood levels but many have found that perfectly normal TSH does not preclude abnormalities of the thyroid. For that matter a patient with normal T3, T4 and TSH may still have classic thyroid symptoms. It is well known and acknowledged that the blood test for thyroid is not always accurate.

To develop "normal" values, labs take the blood of a number of individuals believed to be healthy and average the results to determine a range. Unhealthy people in the control sample will skew that range. Several years ago doctors considered 250 to be a normal adult cholesterol level but while this number may be average, it isn't necessarily healthy. In time, test values were altered to reflect this changed perception.

Something similar may have occurred with thyroid tests. I have seen enough patients with normal lab values who responded positively to thyroid medication to believe this to be the case. One of my patients had typical low thyroid symptoms, but her TSH, T4, and T3 values were perfectly normal. By treating her low thyroid symptoms, however, and not the lab value of her TSH, she was able to get relief of all of her symptoms. At best, basic laboratory tests are screening devices that provide only a snapshot of what is going on in the body at an instant in time.

TSH Is Not the Only Thyroid Check

Most doctors use the TSH blood test as the only marker for thyroid problems. Until the early 1980's, before this test existed, thyroid problems were diagnosed more by physical symptoms after a complete examination. If the patient's symptoms resolved on thyroid medication, the treatment was continued. This approach has some benefits.

Simple temperature readings are also an indicator of thyroid function. Many doctors will recommend a basal body temperature be taken, the temperature of the body upon awakening but before rising from bed or moving around. Shake down a glass thermometer the night before and place it next to the bed. In the morning, place the thermometer under the armpit and lie still for ten minutes. Do this for two mornings. The most accurate temperature for women is on the second day of the menstrual cycle but any two days can be used. A temperature lower than the range of 97.8 — 98.2 might indicate hypothyroidism while a higher reading could suggest hyperthyroidism.

Iodine Patch Test

Another test involves painting a one-inch patch of common drug store iodine on the inner thigh and observing how quickly it absorbs. The iodine should last 24 hours. If it does not, you may be low in iodine and need a supplement. Iodine is necessary for the thyroid to work properly and it is why iodine has been added to our salt. In theory, since everyone eats salt, everyone gets iodine to make the thyroid gland function. Recently, however, we have become afraid of salt due to blood pressure concerns. If salt is not a regular part of the diet, another source of iodine must be used. Kelp is an option and can be taken as a nutritional supplement. The supplement Iodoral is another option. Iodine can be prescribed or SSKI can be purchased at a health food store. (See: Brownstein, David. *Iodine: Why You Need It, Why You Can't Live Without It.*

Patient Is the Best Test

The best thyroid test however is the actual patient and the reported problems. Years ago I saw a boy who appeared exceptionally depressed. He had a pronounced, flat affect. His face was so void of expression he did not even have smile or frown lines on his face. He had no energy and could not jump to get both feet off the floor at one time. His mother was a nurse and felt he had a thyroid problem. For years, she asked doctors to do a simple thyroid test on her son. All refused.
When the child was born, a thyroid test was performed and it indicated low thyroid. However, a few days later a second test came back normal. Ten years later, doctors continued to ignore the child's symptoms and ignored the mother's concerns. I performed a thyroid test on the boy and it came back normal.

As an osteopathic physician, I was taught to treat the patient not just the test results. Although tests can be important and helpful in diagnosing and treating patients, they should be used in the context of other assessments and information. Too often "standard" testing does not reveal the presence of thyroid problems and doctors leave it at that.

I did a clinical trial of thyroid medication with the boy. The results were incredible. Over a short period of time he began to have facial expressions. His parents reported that he had much more energy, no longer seemed depressed and began doing better in school.

I prescribed T3 to him and I told his mother that sometimes administering T3 gives the thyroid gland the boost it needs to work properly without medicine in the future. After several months, I suggested that we try slowly removing the thyroid medicine to see if he could function on his own. His mother began to cry. She felt that this small amount of medicine had given her child his life back. She did not want to take it away from him. He has remained on the thyroid medication and continued to do well.

You might be asking yourself what is the difference between a clinical trial of thyroid medication and a clinical trial of an antidepressant? This young man had normal thyroid lab values, but he also had many of the physical signs of hypothyroidism. Physical signs are different than subjective psychological symptoms.

How Did The Insurance Company React?

Ironically, when the mother tried to get her insurance company to cover the child's thyroid medication, she was refused. Insurance companies are usually quick to pay for psychiatric medicine based on a purely subjective diagnosis but were not willing to pay for treatment of a medical problem. With much determination, the mother packed a lunch and some books to read and drove to the insurance company's office, which was, fortunately, in her hometown.

She asked to see the president of the company. When she was refused, she told the receptionist that she would just sit there and wait until he would see her. She stayed there most of the day until the president finally relented. She explained the situation and the president approved the payment. Sometimes it may take that kind of perseverance to get your insurance company to cover your medical needs.

Drug Companies Also Influence Thyroid Treatments

As with the other medical conditions previously discussed, the pharmaceutical companies also greatly influence the treatment of thyroid disorders. The natural version of the thyroid hormone cannot be patented so drug manufacturers have produced chemical versions. Even though T3 is the active form of thyroid, the version most doctors prescribe contains only T4. Even patients who have had their thyroid removed get only T4. Apparently the belief is that the T4 will sufficiently convert to T3 in the body. However, one study found that decreased T3 can affect the entire body adversely, causing such symptoms as depression, fatigue, myalgia, arthralgia, and cognitive problems. It can also cause a decrease blood flow to the brain and alter carbohydrate metabolism. Low T3 can also decrease serotonin which is thought to be a cause of depression and it can alter the number of adrenal hormone receptor sites. (PR Health Sci J)

According to another study, more than 40% of depressed patients are not helped after taking two trials of antidepressant medications. This study showed that T3 alone improved depression scores in 24.7% of those individuals after only 14 weeks. (Am J Psychiatry)

It has always seemed to me that we should give the patient both the T3 and the T4 or only T3 since it is the active form of thyroid and is available as Cytomel. There are many brands for T4, one of the most common being Synthroid. A few years ago it was discovered that although millions of Americans were taking Synthroid, the FDA had never approved it. Once this information became public, I would have thought that the drug would be immediately pulled from the market but that was not the case. The company was allowed to go through the FDA approval process while still selling the drug. The standard set by the FDA itself should have mandated the removal of the drug and a thorough testing process. Was this an instance of pressure by the pharmaceutical industry? Quite possibly.

The Uniqueness of the Individual

While many doctors argue that a natural combination of T3 and T4 is not accurately delivered in the body, I have not found this to be the case and prefer to try this treatment approach first. These combination drugs are available as Armour Thyroid or Thyrolar and are consistent from pill to pill. Giving someone a prescription with T3 in it assures they will get the active ingredient for their thyroid to work. However, it is also important to realize that the efficacy of thyroid medication varies with individuals. Deciding on dosage and medication type may take several attempts.

My medical training emphasized the uniqueness of the individual. Listening to the patient and taking into account their physical symptoms is as important to the diagnosis as interpreting lab values. "Treat the patient, not the lab value" was a common saying among my professors. When it comes to thyroid problems, that concept seems to have fallen by the wayside. When I see a patient who has been diagnosed with depression, the first thing I do is evaluate their thyroid.

Adrenal Fatigue

Adrenal fatigue can make one feel depressed. The adrenal glands sit on top of the kidneys and produce cortisol when the body is under stress. This should be a short-term reaction but unfortunately today we live in a constantly stressful world that causes these glands to overwork and to become fatigued. To correct this imbalance in the body some people will actually engage in intense activities that help them to generate more cortisol. In addition, adrenal fatigue causes improper thyroid function as well as imbalances in estrogen, progesterone and testosterone. There are many cases of women who exercise to excess and stop having menstrual cycles.

One patient told me that the only way he felt good was to exercise to excess. Every day he ran or did some form of extreme exercise that forced his adrenals to release cortisol and to give him the short-term euphoria known as "Runner's High." In the long-term, however, this strategy would cause even further depletion of his adrenal function. If he continued on his exhausting course, he would need to exercise more and more to achieve the same feeling. What he needed to learn to do was relax, not run even harder.

Understanding Cortisone

Although adrenal fatigue can be treated with low doses of hydrocortisone, many people fear using it as a medical treatment. When cortisone was first discovered and used by the medical profession, it was prescribed in high doses for allergies and arthritis that tremendously relieved the patients' symptoms but carried serious side effects.

High dose cortisone used over a long period of time can cause osteoporosis, ulcers, cataracts, glaucoma, menstrual irregularities, and diabetes. It can suppress growth in children, decrease carbohydrate tolerance, impair wound healing, and suppress the immune system. I saw a young boy in my office with severe arthritis symptoms. He had been treated with high dose cortisone for many years. Even after the medication had been stopped, he did not gain weight or height. In his case cortisone helped the pain of his arthritis but it did not "fix" it and caused new problems with his development.

The use of low dose, or physiological doses of cortisol, needs to be examined more closely. The term "physiological doses" means the dose of the medication is just enough to replace what the body no longer makes. It is not a treatment in the same sense that we think of a medical treatment for a disease but rather a replacement for what the body no longer produces. There are many examples of this in medicine including insulin replacement in diabetes, hormone replacement therapy (HRT) in menopausal women, and of course, thyroid replacement.

Cortisone has been found to be safe even in high doses, when used carefully for a short period of time. It has also been found to be safe when given in the correct physiological dose to those individuals with malfunctioning adrenal glands as explained by William Jeffries, MD in *Safe Uses of Cortisone*. (1996) Jeffries found that correct, physiological doses of cortisol might even fix problems the higher dose could cause.

Just Because You're Depressed

Chapter 5
It's Not Depression, It's De' Hormones
or
Are Your Hormones Driving You Crazy?

A woman's hormones change dramatically while she is pregnant. It should come as no surprise that the hormones would change dramatically again after the baby is delivered. This hormonal imbalance is often referred to as Postpartum Depression. However, this condition is not, as is commonly believed, a psychiatric disorder. It is a hormonal imbalance.

One young woman told me she felt terribly depressed for a year after she had her baby. She said she knew she had no reason to feel that way. She was blessed with a wonderful family and home life but she could not overcome her melancholy. I recommended that she take a 30-day saliva hormone test, which indicated she was low in progesterone. A simple over-the-counter natural progesterone cream applied daily to her skin resulted in the complete cessation of the depressed feelings.

The connection between feeling depressed and hormone problems is very strong. I have seen many women in my practice who became depressed soon after a significant hormonal change. A common story is that shortly after starting menstruation in their teens these women began feeling depressed. Many of these women have been prescribed different antidepressants over the years. None fixed their symptoms and in some instances the drugs made them feel worse.

How Hormones Cause Problems

Women go through a variety of hormone fluctuations throughout their lives. Levels surge during the onset of puberty and then rise and fall in response to the many changes in a woman's life from monthly menstrual cycles and the use of hormonal birth control products to pregnancy and delivery, nursing, peri-menopause and menopause. Through it all, the human body strives to achieve perfect balance.

The most common behavioral symptoms of hormone imbalance are mood swings (including anxiety and depression), fatigue, and nervousness. But hormone imbalances can also cause adrenal stress, insomnia, hair loss, hypoglycemia, headaches, weight gain, breast and cervical cancer as well as thyroid dysfunction, any one of which can be life altering or threatening.

Through such symptoms the body signals malfunctions and gives both the patient and the doctors an opportunity to fix the problem. However, if the doctor prescribes a psychiatric drug to cover the symptoms rather than treating the hormonal imbalance, the woman remains at risk for a variety of health problems.

PMS - Premenstrual Syndrome

Fluctuating hormones during a woman's menstrual cycle cause a host of symptoms called Premenstrual Syndrome. Types and severity of symptoms vary but most commonly include: depression, bloating, headaches, irritability, weight gain, skin problems, cramps, anxiety, mood swings, aggression, fatigue, breast tenderness, and poor concentration. These symptoms can occur in the two weeks before and through the first few days of menstruation.

Women respond in uniquely individual ways to their own hormones throughout their monthly cycle. The same hormone levels that may plague one woman with such symptoms as anger, depression and migraines will not cause any symptoms in another. Women should never allow a doctor to discount their personal symptoms. There are many tests to help identify hormonal fluctuations and to allow for treatment tailored to the individual's specific body levels in order to stabilize those levels and to improve both the symptoms and the woman's overall health.

Menopause

Many times women with menopause or peri-menopause receive either high levels of non-bio-compatible estrogens such as Premarin or psychiatric drugs like antidepressants to control their uncomfortable and life-altering symptoms. Both drugs expose women to equally serious and even life-threatening side effects and do not address or help the underlying health problem.

Menopause is not just about the reduced level of estrogen in the body. The ovaries produce other hormones that diminish with menopause. To simply prescribe estrogen-type drugs to a woman ignores this fact and further disrupts the body's delicate balance.

Estrogen and Estrogen Dominance

Estrogen is a potent and potentially dangerous hormone when not balanced by adequate progesterone. Dr. John Lee, the first to identify and to name this "estrogen dominance," describes unopposed estrogen as a potential cause of cancer in the uterus and of the breast. Estrogen dominance can not only result from taking a hormone prescription but also when estrogen produced by the body is still relatively higher than the levels of progesterone. (Lee & Hopkins, 1996.)

I have a 60-year-old patient whose uterus and ovaries were removed when she was 42. She stopped taking all hormone replacement therapy at 50. Even with no ovaries, testing showed that her estrogen levels were a great deal higher than her progesterone levels. She is now taking a natural, over-the counter progesterone cream that she rubs on her skin each day to balance out the estrogen.

The Importance of Progesterone

Progesterone, in balance, can have numerous benefits to the body. It affects every tissue in the body including the reproductive system, immune system and even the brain. It is known to fight depression, to increase sexual libido, to reduce hot flashes, to improve mental focus, to enhance weight loss, and more. Long-term imbalances of the hormone can result in breast, uterine and ovarian cancer, ovarian cysts and uterine fibroids as well as fibrocystic breast disease.

The symptoms I often see in my office from women low in progesterone are migraine and other headaches (especially before menstruation and during the PMS period), moodiness, depression, excessive bleeding and painful breasts. Women taking natural, bio-identical progesterone report a new feeling of wellbeing.

I take a long and thorough history on my patients – a fifteen-page form for adults. If I am going to help the patient I need to know when their symptoms started and what was going on in their lives at that time. My goal is to try to find the underlying cause of the symptoms so that the problem can be fixed, not just covered up with drugs. When I ask these women, "When did your depressed symptoms start?" followed by "When did you start having periods?" the dates coincide time and time again. From there I evaluate the woman's hormone levels and with appropriate treatment, can often fix or improve the symptoms.

In my opinion, prescribing an antidepressant to these women without a thorough history and a physical exam with appropriate lab work should be considered malpractice. Instead, it's considered "Standard of Care." Listening to a person's symptoms and prescribing an antidepressant is not practicing good medicine. To me it's just lazy medicine.

Medical Research for Women

Women have taken a back seat to men in medical research for years. For a long time, there were no studies performed with women. Professional researchers regarded the practice as justifiable due to the effect fluctuating hormones have on the reliability of physiological research data. Think about that. Until recently there were almost no drugs on the market that are prescribed to women that have been adjusted to or developed to work with the unique physiology of a woman's body. Some drugs were never studied on women at all.

Hormones and the Fountain of Youth

Even in the absence of appropriate studies, doctors had no problem prescribing drugs to women, especially Hormone Replacement Therapy (HRT). The idea of replacing women's decreasing levels of estrogen started many years ago. It was discovered that estrogen from the urine of pregnant horses could modify many symptoms of menopause, especially hot flashes. This Pregnant Mare Urine was named Premarin. Doctors prescribed it to thousands of women.

Although natural estrogen was easy to produce and safer to use, the pregnant mare urine form could be patented by the drug manufacturer and marketed. A doctor, supported by a drug company that produced an estrogen-like medication, wrote a book about this wonderful new product. It was hailed as "The Fountain of Youth" for women. (Wilson, R., 1966) Since no studies had been done, it was not until the numbers of uterine cancer cases in women began to rise that the link was made back to horse urine estrogen and to the dangers of administering estrogen unbalanced by progesterone.

In response, a patented, synthetic form of progesterone called progestin and marketed as Provera was produced to be used as a companion to the horse urine estrogen. Although bio-chemically different from the progesterone made by the human body, the company announced Provera would protect against uterine cancer.

Doctors told their patients they needed to take the hormones even if they were not having menopausal symptoms. Many doctors automatically prescribed hormones to all female patients over fifty. The standard HRT therapy became Premarin and Provera. The news media reported the benefits of this combination. We were told the two hormones were cardiac protective. We were told they were cancer protective. The "fountain of youth" claims resurfaced. (Gregg, V., 2003)

I was not surprised to discover these reports to be untrue. In fact the combination HRT generated the exact opposite results. It did not protect women from cancer or heart disease but it did increase their risks for breast, uterine, ovarian cancers, heart attacks, strokes and dementia. (Women's Health Initiative, July 17, 2002)

The reaction of the medical community to these adverse side effects was interesting to watch. I even heard a doctor on a local television news show say, "If these hormones cause ovarian cancer, we should just take out women's ovaries." After years of prescribing these drugs to their patients, doctors were not prepared to accept their own culpability for the cancers and heart disease from which these individuals suffered.

Many women told me they discontinued the hormones immediately, which was not the best thing to do. They soon found themselves suffering once again from hot flashes, insomnia and irritability. Others told me they decided that since they had not gotten cancer, had a stroke or a heart attack, they would continue with the drugs. Still, sales of HRT fell.

So, if women weren't going to take Premarin and Provera, the pharmaceutical companies offered up a quick replacement – antidepressants. Quickly perceived as the new miracle drug, these pills were dispensed to women who felt depressed without their hormones, had hot flashes, or couldn't sleep. I know one woman who was prescribed an antidepressant for back pain and another who received the drug for diarrhea.

The women who stopped their HRT and began taking the antidepressants may very well have jumped from the frying pan into the fire. Pharmaceutical companies are not required to publish negative results but even if they are not forthcoming with complete product information, you should read the information sheets and seek out other available sources of information. You must take responsibility for yourself and decide if the potential side effects of a drug are worth it. Nearly every drug used to treat depression has a potential life-threatening side effect. See side effects in Appendix II

Don't put yourself blindly into the hands of doctors. According to the FDA, less than 1% of doctors know the side effects of the drugs they prescribe. Some doctors have claimed they don't have time to read the drug warnings. (Neergaard, L., 2002) I'd like to know what they think is more important than taking the time to understand the potential side effects of the drugs they are handing out.

I am a cynic when it comes to medicine. I've heard too many horror stories from my patients and had too many personal and familial experiences to be a blind believer. I recognize the limits of medicine and see the control the drug companies have over the way a doctor practices medicine. I am aware that most doctors do not know the side effects of the drugs they prescribe and that the FDA allows the drug company representatives to make decisions concerning the approval of their drugs. The consumers are not being well protected nor are they being well informed about alternate treatments. In the instance of the controversy about HRT, television and magazine reports talked at length about Premarin and Provera but I never heard anyone discuss bio-identical hormones.

Bio-Identical Hormones

Bio-identical hormones are well named, as they are bio-chemically identical to those naturally occurring in the human body. Women should know that these hormones are available and that when they are prescribed properly they can relieve menopausal symptoms. Bio-identical hormones are made to look identical to our own natural hormones. If they look the same, they should act the same and they should go to the same receptor sites. Premarin and Provera have no bio-chemical similarity to our own hormones. Even with bio-identical hormones, it is important to have the proper balance.

We have known for years that estrogen can cause breast cancer. It was also assumed, without any valid research, that estrogen was protective for heart disease and HRT was being pushed for that purpose. I attended an educational meeting given by a gynecologist who was adamant that women of menopause age should be taking HRT. He said, "Women don't want to take HRT because it increases the risk of breast cancer, but HRT decreases the risk of heart disease and heart disease is more prevalent in women than breast cancer."

It concerned me greatly that this gynecologist thought he could make this choice for women and I was angered that he made the statement without an ounce of corroborating evidence. Because post-menopausal women are more prone to heart disease, decreased estrogen was assumed to be the culprit. When researchers studied the effects of estrogen they used the horse urine form, not the bio-identical. The results confirmed the dangers of the horse urine estrogen and when combined with progestins, it did increase the risk of breast cancer as well as that for heart disease, stroke and pulmonary embolism.

On the other hand, in his book *What Your Doctor May Not Tell You About Women's Breast Cancer*, (2004) Dr. John Lee reported observing hundreds of women in his practice who had not been diagnosed with breast cancer. All used bio-identical progesterone cream that Lee believed to be protecting his patients from cancer. Most doctors, however, know little or nothing about bio-identical hormones and the drug companies like it that way as these substances offer no profit potential to the industry. (Lee, 2004)

Progesterone vs. Progestins

Progestins, like Provera, do not resemble at all the bio-chemical structure of a woman's natural progesterone. They cannot be taken during pregnancy without risking serious consequences for the fetus. Because of this many doctors also assume that bio-identical progesterone is toxic as well.

A woman needs progesterone to carry a pregnancy to term. Many women who cannot become pregnant are simply deficient in real progesterone. I know of a case in which the doctor prescribed Premarin for a woman trying to have a baby. This treatment would further increase her estrogen dominance making it even more difficult for her to conceive. By the same token, I know of cases in which birth control pills, which are usually made with synthetic estrogens, shut down the ovaries and it took months or even years for the ovaries to recover.

Andrea Yates Gets a Retrial

Andrea Yates, a Houston woman convicted of drowning her five children, received repeated diagnoses of post-partum depression. She saw several psychiatrists, was hospitalized, and took many psychiatric drugs – often in combination – including antidepressants and anti-psychotic medications.

At the time of the drownings, Yates had been prescribed Effexor, Remeron, Haldol and Wellbutrin, all psychiatric drugs. (Fecher, L., 2002) If four such drugs were required, one cannot help but wonder how effective they are and the side effects of the medications to the nervous system – as reported by the manufacturers – are staggering:

> Remeron: May impair judgment, abnormal thinking, confusion, apathy, anxiety, agitation, delirium, delusions, depersonalization, hallucinations, manic reaction, hostility, emotional lability, paranoid reaction, psychotic depression.

> Effexor: Abnormal thinking, agitation, confusion, depersonalization, depression, and anxiety.

> Wellbutrin: Impaired sleep, hostility, delusions, agitation, anxiety, confusion, euphoria, and sensory disturbance.

> Haldol: Agitation, anemia, anxiety, blurred vision, confusion, epileptic seizures, exaggerated feeling of well-being, hallucinations, headache, involuntary movements, stupor, sleeplessness, sluggishness, vertigo, visual problems.

Each of these drugs can cause severe neurological symptoms. If each, in isolation, could cause symptoms that could have put Yates in a condition to murder her children (hallucinations, abnormal thinking, delusions, etc.), what would the four in combination do? The medications have never been tested together. What were the prescribing doctors thinking? With no adequate understanding of the potential for cascading side effects with these medications, I cannot help but question the original guilty verdict in the Yates trial.

Understand, I do not condone Yates' actions, but the entire focus of the trial was unfortunate for her. I believe her physicians bear much of the responsibility for this tragedy. According to newspaper reports, the mental health community used the Yates trial to educate the public about mental illness. They hoped to show the public Yates needed treatment for her postpartum depression. They felt she was not responsible for what she did because she was mentally ill. Her attorney used insanity as her defense. (Jarvis, J., 2002)

That defense may have kept her from being executed, but it did not prevent the guilty verdict and subsequent 40-year sentence. If the mental health community believed Yates was not guilty because of mental illness, it had an opportunity to help her – an eight-year opportunity. Shortly after the birth of her first child in 1994, Yates told her doctor, "Satan told her to get a knife and stab someone." (Brooks, K., 2002) Not only did her doctors not help Yates, her condition worsened under their care. To me, the mental health community showed the world how truly incompetent it can be.

During a June 1999 hospitalization Yates was prescribed Zoloft which, according to Pfizer, can cause psychosis and agitation. Her doctor increased the dosage three-fold in only four days. According to the drug manufacturer it should not be increased more often than once each week. (Jarvis)

When Yates was hospitalized again in July 1999 she received Zoloft, Zyprexa, Cogentin, Haloperidol, Lorazepam, diphenhydramine, Wellbutrin and Effexor. According to the medical record summary, these drugs appear to have been "mixed and matched" with Yates receiving as many as five different drugs at one time. She was discharged from the hospital with prescriptions for Wellbutrin, Effexor, Haldol and Cogentin. During a third hospitalization in March 2001 records indicate Yates was prescribed Effexor, Wellbutrin, Risperdal, Cogentin and Restoril and was discharged with prescriptions for Risperdal, Effexor and Wellbutrin. (Jarvis)

Following her conviction Yates continued to receive psychiatric drugs in prison. (Jarvis) I would be interested to know her hormone levels. Since she has not been pregnant for several years, the levels may have evened out some but I suspect they are still abnormal. How tragic that Yates' body cried out with classic symptoms of postpartum hormone imbalance but no doctor treated her for that specific problem. We will never know how her life and the lives of her children would have been different if her physicians had followed that course of treatment.

Andrea Yates did get a new trial. I am glad she was found "Not guilty by reason of insanity". From what I have read, I do not believe Andrea Yates was "insane" due to post-partum depression. I do believe she was made "insane" by the psychiatrists who placed her on these drugs.

I hoped someone introduces the concept that she may have had a hormone imbalance. If all the facts and information relating to her medical treatment – or mistreatment – were entered into evidence those eight years of psychiatric prescribing would be placed under close and perhaps unfavorable scrutiny. If doctors begin to look for the true underlying causes of the symptoms of depression instead of reflexively handing out antidepressants, great strides could be made to prevent any other woman and her family from going through what Andrea Yates and her children experienced.

Although much less tragic in its consequences, I also found the media debate about Tom Cruise and Brooke Shields to be very interesting. Brooke Shields has spoken openly about taking antidepressants after the birth of her first child. She told the media she had been diagnosed with Post-partum Depression and reported that she was grateful for the relief the medication gave her. Tom Cruise indicated his concern for her use of antidepressants. He told Matt Lauer of *The Today Show* that "I really care about Brooke Shields. I think, here is a wonderful and talented woman. And I want to see her do well. And I know psychiatry is a pseudo-science. . . . The thing I am saying about Brooke is that there's misinformation, OK? And she doesn't understand the history of psychiatry."

Much discussion followed from the media. I think it was an important topic to be discussed. It started people talking about the subject. What I found to be most interesting, however, was that every one of the "experts" that were interviewed on television or for the newspapers or magazines, said that Post-partum Depression was a real disease.

They went on to say that it was real because women have real hormonal changes after giving birth. I was quite surprised to hear them say this. If women's symptoms were caused from a hormone imbalance, why were they calling it Post-partum Depression? They should be diagnosing it as Post Partum Hormone Imbalance or Hormone Deficiency.

If a woman were to receive the correct diagnosis she could then be given the correct treatment, bio-identical hormones, instead of labeling her with a psychiatric diagnosis and prescribing antidepressants. To me the way Brooke Shields and Andrea Yates were diagnosed and treated makes as much sense as diagnosing depression in someone with diabetes and then prescribing an antidepressant instead of insulin.

PMDD

In addition to the postpartum depression label women must also face having their premenstrual symptoms categorized as a psychological malady, Premenstrual Dysphoric Disorder or PMDD. According to the DSM the symptoms of PMDD are:

> Markedly depressed mood, marked anxiety, marked affective lability and decreased interest in activities. These symptoms have regularly occurred during the last week of the luteal phase in most menstrual cycles during the past year. The symptoms begin to remit within a few days of the onset of menses (the follicular phase) and are always absent in the week following menses. (APA, 2000, p. 771)

These symptoms clearly reflect a hormone imbalance. Why would anyone have a psychiatric disorder once a month? Yet commercials paid for by Eli Lilly bombard women with statements like, "Call your doctor to find out if Sarafem is right for you for the treatment of PMDD." Remember, Sarafem is actually Prozac produced under a new name.

Eli Lilly spends millions of dollars not just promoting their drug but also the so-called disorder they claim Sarafem treats. Given the relationship drug companies and their representatives cultivate with doctors, including "educational" seminars, new drugs and new disorders easily become a part of the mentality of the medical community in perfectly matched pairs. In the absence of this carefully crafted marketing scheme women currently labeled as suffering from PMDD would be accurately diagnosed with a hormone deficiency and treated accordingly.

The DSM goes on to say:

> Some individuals with general medical conditions may present with dysphoria (restlessness) and fatigue that are exacerbated during the premenstrual period. Examples include seizure disorders, thyroid and other endocrine disorders, cancer,

> systemic lupus erythematosus, anemia, endometriosis and various infections. Attempts should be made to distinguish these general medical conditions from premenstrual dysphoric disorder by history, laboratory testing, or physical exam. (APA, 2000, p. 771)

Based on this information it would seem that the Sarafem ad should say, "See your doctor to find out if you have any medical condition causing your symptoms." Although the DSM acknowledges that medical conditions cause the symptoms and recommends physical exams, lab work, and a clear understanding of the patient's history, these things rarely happen. If the "PMDD" patients I see are any indication, these things *never* happen.

Unfortunately it's not just psychiatrists handing out the pills or making the psychiatric diagnoses. Patients must take responsibility for their own treatment and insure that this does not happen. No one should be prescribed an antidepressant without a complete physical exam and thorough medical evaluation.

How Bad Drugs Lead To More Bad Drugs

In addition to automatically prescribing HRT for women over fifty, doctors also like to prescribe calcium to this age group to protect them from osteoporosis. This is not necessarily the best approach. (Sanson, 2003)

When women receive Premarin and calcium together the combination can cause some harmful side effects. By placing women in an estrogen dominant state the Premarin raises the likelihood for depression and the estrogen and calcium block the uptake of magnesium, which in turn also can cause depression. Once a woman reports these feelings she's often given an antidepressant. One wrong treatment leads to a second.

A hormone imbalance and a nutritional deficiency aren't the makings of a psychiatric disorder. Had the correct hormone been given in the first place, perhaps bio-identical progesterone, the women most likely would not have reported depressed feelings at all. The problem is not depression, but de-hormones.

Just Because You're Depressed

Chapter 6
Magnesium and Other Nutrients
or
A Simple Nutrient Could Save your Life

While searching the medical literature for a link between depression and magnesium deficiency I found many articles connecting the two. Previously in my own practice I used magnesium to treat asthma, migraine headaches, muscle aches and pain. Several patients also reported that their depressed feelings vanished when taking the supplement. My subsequent research yielded many articles establishing the link between magnesium depletion and depression.

Magnesium, the Magnificent Mineral

More than 350 biochemical processes require the nutrient magnesium. Referred to as the body's natural tranquilizer, magnesium helps to relax the nerves, muscles, bronchial tubes, and blood vessels. Deficiencies can cause depression, asthma, cramps, calcification of small arteries, EKG changes, migraines and other headaches, kidney stones, muscles weakness, muscle tremors, muscle tics, heart attacks, neuromuscular problems, PMS and vertigo. Additional deficiency symptoms may include agitation and anxiety, twitching and other muscle spasm and weakness, insomnia, irritability, nausea and vomiting, abnormal heart rhythms, confusion, hyperventilation and even seizures. (Brown, et al, 1999)

Studies done with depressed patients discovered low plasma magnesium levels that began to normalize during recovery. In some individuals, treatment with intravenous magnesium led to faster improvement of their condition. (Frizel D., et al, 1969) In a trial with 32 women suffering from PMS symptoms a 360mg a day dose of magnesium on day fifteen of their cycle to the onset of menstruation was more effective than a placebo in relieving mood changes. Since dietary surveys show that Americans do not get the recommended daily allowance for magnesium, a nutritional supplement of 200-400mg a day may help many people with their feelings of depression. (Facchinetti, F., et al, 1991; Morgan, K., et al, 1985; Singh, A., et al, 1989)

In addition to helping with the conditions already cited, magnesium depletion has been found to be an underlying cause of many other medical disorders, including allergies, chronic fatigue, cardiac arrhythmias, diabetes, hyperactivity, premenstrual symptoms, cancer, high blood pressure, seizures, high cholesterol, high triglycerides, osteoporosis, stroke, Alzheimer's, hormone abnormalities, and decreased immune system function. As with thyroid problems, there is a clear association with magnesium and many different so-called psychiatric disorders. Magnesium has even been referred to as "Nature's Valium."

Magnesium Depletion

The causes of magnesium depletion are many: pregnancy, lactation, calcium ingestion, alcohol, estrogen, kidney dysfunction, stress, chronic disease, pain, diabetes, gastrointestinal problems, hyperthyroidism, diuretics, and as a side effect of a number of medications. I believe that most Americans are deficient in magnesium and the medical literature supports this supposition. If everyone currently hospitalized in this country received a shot of magnesium, I suspect we could empty half the beds.

Just eating a balanced diet is not likely to keep enough magnesium in the body, much less all the other nutrients we need for good health. I have heard many doctors say, "If you eat a balanced diet, you don't need to take nutritional supplements." I am not convinced that anyone really knows what a balanced diet consists of and even if we did know, I doubt many individuals would eat accordingly.

There are several different methods for evaluating magnesium deficiency. The "gold standard" method involves the patient collecting urine for 24 hours, receiving one or two injections of magnesium depending on body weight, and collecting urine for another 24 hours. The goal is to see how much magnesium the body keeps which in turns indicates how much it needs. Analyzing the levels of magnesium excreted before and after the injections allows for the mathematical computation of the amount of injected magnesium retained. Retention of more than 20% is considered magnesium depletion. Blood tests are not an accurate picture of the levels of useful magnesium in the body.

Magnesium Supplements

In my experience taking oral magnesium will help keep the levels from falling further but I am not convinced that supplements will bring a low level back to normal. When one of my patients is particularly deficient, I recommend intravenous treatment or injections for a few weeks. Many of my patients feel so good while taking the shots they ask if they can continue. I have found that the patient is the best judge of when to stop the shots or when to return for more.

Depression and Other Nutrients

A patient of mine went to see her regular doctor with a complaint of feeling depressed. The doctor did no lab work or physical exam. Instead, he just listened to her symptom, depression, and prescribed Effexor, an antidepressant. She was uncomfortable with this and did not want to take the prescribed drug, so she came to see me instead. I did a blood test and found that she was anemic. Her iron level was extremely low. Treatment with iron shots relieved her symptom of depression.

Depression has also been linked to folic acid deficiency. Researchers from Tufts University studied 3,000 ethnically diverse subjects ranging in age from fifteen to 39 with no depression to chronic symptoms. Blood tests showed that the depressed individuals had folate serum concentrations lower than those with no depression. The lead researcher, Martha Morris, Ph.D. concluded, "Folate supplementation may be indicated during the year following a depressive episode." (Morris, 2003).

In similar studies depressed patients were found to have inadequate levels of pyridoxine or Vitamin B6, which is necessary for the conversion of tryptophan into serotonin, a neurotransmitter that, when deficient, is believed to cause depression. (Werbach, M.) Neurotransmitters are those elements in the body that conduct chemical messages. Many antidepressants currently on the market affect serotonin in the body by keeping it active and preventing it from going back into the nerve to be used again and again. However, if an individual does not have the vitamin B6 needed to make serotonin, the antidepressant may make the person feel even worse by disrupting the natural production process. Both estrogen and oral contraceptives can deplete the body's supply of B6.

Vitamin C deficiency has always been associated with scurvy, which first manifests itself as depression. Studies have shown that 32% of patients in psychiatric hospitals registered low levels of Vitamin C and that such individuals may be in a "sub-scurvy" state calling for ascorbic acid (Vitamin C) supplementation. (Am J Clin Nutrition, 1971)

Other research has linked depression to Vitamin B12 deficiency and to severe obesity. (BMC Psychiatry, 2003; Archives of Internal Medicine, 2003) Other nutrient deficiencies that have been shown to affect depression are iron, omega-6 fatty acids, biotin, copper and potassium. Also found to be associated with depression are 5-HTP, the immediate precursor to serotonin, hypericin (the active ingredient in St. John's Wort), SAMe and L-tryptophan (another precursor to serotonin). (Werbach, M.)

The most commonly used serotonin precursor is 5-HTP

As early as 1957, references show that scientists had determined that 5-HTP could be used to increase serotonin levels. (J Biol Chem, 1957; J Clin Invest, 1957) Many studies have examined the ability of 5-HTP to increase serotonin levels and reduce the symptoms associated with low serotonin. The general finding is that 5-HTP will increase serotonin levels, that it is more effective than a placebo, and can be as effective as prescription medication in some patients. (Van Praag, H., 1982)

Tryptophan-Serotonin Pathway

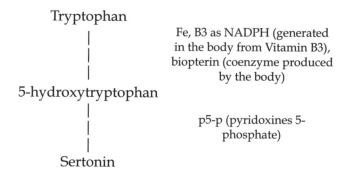

Tryptophan

Fe, B3 as NADPH (generated in the body from Vitamin B3), biopterin (coenzyme produced by the body)

5-hydroxytryptophan

p5-p (pyridoxines 5-phosphate)

Sertonin

Serotonin is normally synthesized from the amino acid tryptophan. In order for this to occur in the brain, tryptophan must be able to cross the blood-brain barrier.

Disrupting the Body's Serotonin

Studies demonstrate the ability of serotonin depletion to reduce the effectiveness of serotonin-acting antidepressants. (Tryptophan depletion and serotonin loss in selective serotonin reuptake inhibitor-treated depression. Praschak-Rieder N., et al, 2004)

"Overall, these studies agree that an amino acid cocktail devoid of tryptophan will deplete serotonin and that this depletion can cause the symptoms to return in patients being treated with serotonin-acting medications. This information seems so logical. A machine that makes paper clips out of wire won't work without wire so why would a drug that affects a neurotransmitter be effective without the neurotransmitter it works upon?" (Argyropoulos, S.V., et al, 2004)

Neurotransmitters such as serotonin and norepinephrine are constructed in the body from amino acids, vitamins and mineral co-factors. If the body does not have a sufficient supply of these amino acids, it will result in neurotransmitter depletion, which can lead to insufficient or unbalanced neurotransmission with systemic results. Conversely, it would seem that giving these amino acids and vitamin and mineral co-factors would correct the imbalance so no antidepressant prescription would be needed.

Neurotransmitters are fat-soluble and do not cross the blood-brain barrier. When given to a patient orally or by IV they will do nothing to increase neurotransmitters at the site of the problem in the brain. Neurotransmitters are produced on-site in the neurons of the brain from their amino acid precursors which can readily cross the blood-brain barrier. Sufficient amino acids plus vitamin and mineral cofactors must be present to produce sufficient neurotransmitters.

What emerges here is a portrait of depression too complex to simply receive a psychiatric label. With multiple potential factors underlying such symptoms, many nutritional in nature, it seems to me that a far safer approach to treating depression would be to supplement the nutrients and other chemicals the body needs to make its neurotransmitters function effectively rather than further upsetting the balance with inappropriate psychiatric drugs like antidepressants.

The antidepressant manufacturers admit they don't really understand how their Selective Serotonin Re-uptake Inhibitors work, but they have a theory based on the idea that a deficiency of the neurotransmitter serotonin causes depression. (Other neurotransmitters include dopamine, epinephrine, norepinephrine, GABA and histamine.) The drug companies claim that SSRI drugs keep serotonin more active by preventing its "re-uptake" back into the nerve. (PDR, 2006) Basically the drug keeps the existing serotonin in the nerve pathway thus fooling your body into believing more serotonin has been produced.

Although the product inserts do not say these drugs are addictive, many people have trouble getting off an SSRI. Based on the mechanism of the drugs, it appears that the effect of these drugs is to actually deplete the body's supply of serotonin even further. By design the serotonin is supposed to go back into the cell for re-use. While someone taking an SSRI might feel better initially, it has been my experience that most will, in the long term, feel worse and will become dependent on the drug as the body attempts to achieve adequate serotonin function.

A better and more natural way to increase serotonin in the body would be to give the body what it needs to make its own serotonin. Respect the natural process, not disrupt it. The body needs certain nutrients to produce serotonin. Once any medical conditions such as hypothyroidism, adrenal fatigue, hormone deficiencies, allergies or nutritional deficiencies have been corrected, giving the individual the nutrients needed to make serotonin naturally can allow the body to achieve the balance it needs.

Evaluate Nutritional Deficiencies

Anyone with depressed feelings should be evaluated for nutritional deficiencies. Many of these nutrients are water-soluble so they can be taken without concern of over dosing. Anyone can pick up a book on vitamins, minerals and other nutrients at a health food store or bookstore and read more about the benefits of nutritional supplementation. This strategy seeks to restore balance to the body and does not involve masking symptoms with unnecessary psychiatric medications that may, in fact, worsen the patient's condition.

Nutritional Recommendations by Age

Age	2-6	6-12	12 and up
B2 (mg)	5	10	15
B6 (mcg)	10	20	30
B5 (mg)	10	25	50
Folate (mcg)	400	800	1200
Calcium (mg)	100	200	300
Magnesium (mg)	150	300	450
Zinc (mg)	5	10	15
DMAE (mg)	100	150	200
DHA (mg)	100	100	100

Beta Carotene (IU)	3500	7,000	10,500
Vitamin C (mg)	250	500	1000
Vitamin E (IU)	100	200	300
Evening Primrose Oil (mg)	500	500	500
Chromium (mcg)	30	60	90

Chapter 7
Allergies
Or
Depression Is Nothing to Sneeze At

Neuropsychologist Paul Marshall maintains that unless a person's allergies are treated, depression will remain and that allergies are often overlooked by psychotherapists as a cause of depression. This does not surprise me as psychotherapists are not physicians and would not have the medical training to alert them to the presence of or consequences of allergies. However, psychiatrists *are* physicians, so they should know to look for these medical conditions. Marshall writes that those with allergies and depression should get allergy shots or avoid their allergens. "If not, they may never recover fully from either." (Marshall P.S., et al, 2002)

There are many references in the medical literature to an association between depression and allergies. So many references, in fact, that it really shocks me that more doctors do not evaluate their patients for allergies before labeling them with depression and prescribing antidepressants.

Antidepressants Were First Antihistamines

The first antidepressants produced were actually formulated from antihistamines. That should be a big clue that there is a real association between the two problems. These antidepressants are the tricyclic antidepressants, such as Tofranil (Imipramine), Norpramin, Anafranil, Elavil, Pamelor, Sinequan and Surmontil. Tricyclic antidepressants are potent antihistamines and this may actually explain why they are so effective as antidepressants. (Richarelson, E., 1982)

When we look at the association in the medical literature, it becomes obvious to me that allergies underlie many if not most depressed symptoms. In 275 patients, their emotional symptoms (such as depression and anxiety) improved when bread, sugar, caffeine and chocolate were eliminated. (Borok, G., 1995)

More than 70% of patients diagnosed with depression had a history of allergy. (Bell, I., et al, 1991) Researchers found a high number of positive IgE antibody tests, which indicate allergies, in depressed individuals. Mold and egg whites were the most often occurring. (Sugerman, A., et al, 1982) In addition, children with severe allergies are more likely to be depressed than children who don't have allergies. (*British Journal of Child Psychology and Psychiatry*) Studies also indicate that patients with clinical depression have higher rates of allergies than those who are not depressed. (*Journal Watch Psychiatry*, 2002)

Foods have been shown to cause a number of mental and behavioral symptoms through different mechanisms including cerebral allergy, food addiction, hypoglycemia, caffeinism, hypersensitivity to food additives, reactions to vasoactive amines in food and reactions to neuropeptides formed from foods. (Rippere V., 1984)

In another study, 33% of depressed people had allergies and only 2% of controls were allergic. (Nasr S., et al, 1981) In yet another study, 85% of depressed children and adults had allergies. (Ossofsky, H.J., 1976)

One might wonder why depression seems to occur in so many individuals who have allergies. The answer is found in basic physiology. According to my freshman medical school physiology textbook, the same cells that release histamine, also release serotonin, the neurochemical thought to be associated with depression. (Guyton, A., 1991)

These histamine and serotonin releasing cells are called mast cells, which are found throughout the body. While most people think of allergies as a runny nose, itchy skin or asthma, mast cells are found every where. They are found in the bladder and can cause bladder spasm and bed wetting. They are found in the muscles and can cause muscle spasm and pain. They are also found in the brain and may cause hyperactivity or depression.

If the first antidepressants were antihistamines, why couldn't we just use antihistamines for the same purpose today? We can perform allergy testing to find out which allergens are causing the depressed symptoms and remove the allergen from our lives or we can treat the allergy with injections.

There are many ways to detect allergies. Blood tests can be performed or skin testing can be done. Many doctors who are not familiar with IgG allergy testing may just test for IgE and when the tests are negative, inform the patient that no allergies are present. However, IgG testing is now discussed in the medical literature especially where gastrointestinal problems are concerned. Also, one study found that children who had IgG allergies to foods when they were young, were more likely to have IgE inhalant allergies when they were older. (Calkoven, 1991)

The other problem with blood tests is that they will not tell you how the allergen makes you feel. You may have many allergies but one may give you a runny nose while another causes you to feel depressed. A blood test is not the best way to get the information you need. Allergy skin testing all the allergens at one time will not get you the information either. The skin testing might show you are allergic, but if all allergens are applied at once, just like the blood test, you will not know which one makes you feel depressed.

The only way to allergy test and to find out which allergen is causing your symptoms is to skin test one allergen at a time. This process takes longer, but you get much more information from it. If you have headaches, asthma or any other symptom, this method can tell you if your condition is caused by allergies and specifically by which allergen.

Once the allergen has been identified, it can be removed from the environment or neutralized with injections. This kind of allergy testing and treatment is called Provocation/Neutralization. Not only does it have the benefit of telling you exactly which allergen is causing the symptoms, but it also treats the symptoms immediately. You do not have to wait for the process of desensitization to occur. Desensitization can take two to three years to become effective. Relief from Provocation/Neutralization is immediate when it is successful.

On my website, www.blockcenter.com there is a video of a young boy undergoing Provocation/Neutralization allergy testing. While testing he has extreme changes in his behavior and his ability to focus and concentrate. This video is a good example of what can happen to the brain when you have an allergy reaction. If allergies can cause this kind of brain changes, they can certainly cause depression.

Depression mechanisms can relate to allergies, inflammation and neurotransmitter depletion. We must evaluate and treat the allergies as well as supply the amino acid precursors (5-HTP) and co-factors p5-p (which supplies the vitamin B6) to hopefully allow the depressed feelings to resolve.

If your allergies are causing you to be depressed, you don't have depression, you have allergies.

Chapter 8
Drug Side Effects
Or
What You Don't Know Can Hurt You

After my own daughter was given Valium and the antidepressant, Tofranil (Imipramine) as treatment for her chronic bladder infections she was sick for three years. Now, that does not surprise me. I know that less than 1% of doctors actually know the side effects of the drugs they prescribe either in a broad sense of the "typical" side effects reported by the manufacturer or in a specific sense given an individual patient's history and genetic make-up.

I can only assume that had my daughter's doctor known the potential side effects of the drugs she received he would at least have monitored her blood levels. And I certainly hope that when he told me to stop the drugs abruptly he did not know that "cold turkey" withdrawal from Valium can be fatal. Ignorance, however, is not an excuse. It was his responsibility to know. I trusted him with my child.

In the same way that doctors are responsible for considering the myriad medical factors that may contribute to symptoms of depression, the pharmaceutical companies are responsible for keeping doctors updated about the potential adverse affects their products pose for patients. Doctors also need to be informed about how to safely discontinue a medication. I feel fortunate that Michelle recovered, although it took many years. Other people have not been so lucky.

Eli Lilly's top selling drug is Zyprexa. (Richards, B., 2006) Though Zyprexa is indicated for psychosis, there are not enough people with that diagnosis to reap the $4.2 billion in sales realized in 2005. Lilly markets the drug as a mood stabilizer for children and teenagers even though it is not indicated for this population. Zyprexa's adverse effects include cardiac arrest and hypotension, Parkinson-like motor impairment, unbearable restlessness, and acute weight gain. According to some sources, Eli Lilly and the FDA covered up twenty deaths and twelve suicides that resulted from the use of Zyprexa. (Richards)

Recently ads for another Eli Lilly drug, Cymbalta, have begun to air on television with the theme "Depression Hurts." While that may be true, the pain felt by the family of 19-year-old Traci Johnson has been just as unbearable. Traci enrolled as a "normal" subject in a clinical trial for Cymbalta after her father lost his job. She needed the $150 to stay in college. She never got the chance to use her earnings. Although she was considered physically and psychologically "normal" prior to the trial, Traci hanged herself in the Eli Lilly laboratory. Bryon Richards, author of the book *Fight for Your Health*, discovered, through the Freedom of Information Act, that 41 deaths and 13 suicides occurred in patients taking Cymbalta. However, the "Important Safety Information" section of the official website for Cymbalta, depressionhurts.com includes the following statement:

> A large study combined results of 24
> different studies of children and teenagers
> with depression or other illnesses, In these
> studies, patients either took a placebo (sugar
> pill) or an antidepressant for 1 to 4 months.
> No one committed suicide in these studies,
> but some patients became
> suicidal." (Cymbalta, Important Safety
> Information, depressionhurts.com)

The Tragedy of Brad Pitan

In 2004 Joe D. Pitan appeared before an FDA advisory panel investigating whether SSRIs increase the risk of suicide in children. (It is also possible that the drugs increase the chance that these children will harm others.) Pitan read a letter from his son who, at the age of 12, experienced these horrific side effects.

Dear FDA, My name is Chris Pitan. I am
now 14 years old. I would like to tell you
what happened to me, what the medication
did to me, and how I felt when I was taking
Zoloft. Because of this medication, I took the
lives of two people that I loved more than
anything, my grandparents." (Cato, J., 2004)

On November 29, 2002 the bodies of Joe Frank and Joy Roberts
Pitan were found in the burned remains of their home. In April
2004 Chris Pitan stood trial, as an adult, for double murder and
arson. (Cato) In 2005 he received a 30 year prison term when
jurors rejected the defense argument that Zoloft drove him to
commit the murders. (Polk, J., 2005)

Chris described in his letter to the FDA how, just days before the
killings, his doctor dramatically increased the dosage of his
medication.

I went to the doctor and he gave me a
sample pack of Zoloft. He told me to take 50
mgs once in the morning and once at night..
. . A week after my doctor gave me a sample
pack, I went back and he gave me two
packs, and he told me to take a 100 mgs once
in the morning and once at night. (Cato)

Forty-eight hours later his grandparents were dead. Pitan, an
unhappy young man living with a father described as a stern
disciplinarian, had run away from home and threatened suicide.
After six days in a Florida psychiatric center his grandparents
took him to their home in South Carolina where a doctor put
Chris on Zoloft to replace a medication he had taken in the
center. Family members reported Pitan became fidgety,
complained of a burning sensation on his skin, and could not sit
still. (Polk)

When Pitan got into a fight with a younger child on the school
bus his grandfather spoke of returning the youth to Florida. The
next night Pitan loaded a shotgun with birdshot walked into his

grandparents' bedroom and killed them. (Polk) Pitan then set the house on fire and fled in his grandfather's truck. (Springer, J., 2005.)

Although the jury did not believe that Zoloft caused Chris Pitan's actions, the drug had never been approved to treat depression in children. (Cato) Subsequent to the verdict in this case the FDA altered its stance on the use of these drugs in children saying they, "increased the risk of suicidal thinking and behavior in short-term studies of adolescents and children" with depression and other psychiatric disorders. (Polk)

The same day Joe Pitan read his letter to the FDA other horror stories were entered into the record. There was the 13-year-old who hanged himself in a closet seven days after starting to take Zoloft and the teen who held a teacher and 23 classmates hostage with a high-powered rifle after a dosage increase of Effexor. Two weeks into treatment with Paxil a Stanford graduate stabbed herself twice in the chest with a butcher's knife and died on her parents' kitchen floor. And finally there was the boy taking Prozac who committed suicide and left behind a note thanking his parents for fourteen wonderful years of life. (Cato) Clearly the full effects of these medications have either not been disclosed or have not been discovered.

Informed Consent

Since more than 99% of doctors do not know the side effects of the drugs they prescribe, they cannot be giving their patients informed consent; information regarding all the potential side effects of a treatment as well as information about all other possible treatments available. It is the doctor's responsibility to inform their patients and when they do not inform them, the doctors are still responsible. However, the patient must protect themselves and obtain the knowledge they need to make an educated decision concerning their own care.

Ask your pharmacist for copies of product information sheets or find the latest edition of *The Physician's Desk Reference* (PDR) at a bookstore. Unlike the printed sheet you receive when picking up a prescription, which contains only partial information, the full product information or the text of the PDR will at least contain as much data regarding side effects and dangers as the drug companies have released. A great deal of this information can also be found by searching the Internet.

However, if drug companies withhold information you are still working with only a partial understanding of any medication. Remember, you are the one who will have to live with the side effects if they occur. You are the one who should make the decision as to whether or not any drug is worth the risk. I have heard many doctors say, "All drugs have side effects. If the patient knew what they were, they wouldn't take any drug." While most drugs have potential side effects, with full information, individuals can make the best decision for themselves.

Unfortunately there are many "ifs" that factor into the administration of drugs in this country. If the drug companies were required to release all information about the drugs . . . if the doctors asked the pharmaceutical representatives about the side effects of their drugs . . . if the doctors read the side effects in the PDR – if these things happened perhaps physicians wouldn't be so quick to prescribe so many drugs to so many people. If doctors had had more education in nutrition, or practiced medicine based on the physiology and biochemistry they learned in medical school, there would not be so many adverse reactions to prescription drugs. But at this point in the evolution of our medical community those statements are still just that, "ifs."

Here are some even bigger "ifs" and a consequence I would like to see come to pass. If the drug companies are allowed to withhold important information from the FDA and doctors and if the FDA allows individuals with a financial conflict of interest to approve a drug for use, the public should be able to easily hold the pharmaceutical companies responsible for problems caused by the use of their drugs.

Prescription Drug Reactions

Medical errors may be the third leading cause of death in the United States. One study found that 106,000 of the 225,000 people who die each year because of medical mistakes do so as a result of adverse reactions to medications. (Starfield) Even using a more conservative figure of 98,000 deaths per year due to medical mistakes, more people die as a result of such error than from highway accidents, breast cancer, or AIDS. (Kohn, et al, 2000) More frightening perhaps is the fact that more than two million hospitalized patients each year experience some level of adverse drug reaction. Of those reactions, 75% could be traced to the apparent toxicity of the drug rather than any kind of allergic reaction. (Jason, et al., 1998)

Potential Adverse Effects from Antidepressants

At the back of this book, in Appendix II, you will find a list of some of the antidepressants and other drugs often prescribed for depression and some of their side effects as reported by the manufacturer. These are only the cardiac and nervous system side effects that appear in the PDR. Many other side effects have been reported.

Drugs Are Not As Good As Their Marketing

I have always wondered why we need so many psychiatric drugs if they actually work as well as the psychiatrists seem to think they do. We've illustrated that these drugs mask but do not fix symptoms and in addition they can themselves affect the central nervous system and cardiovascular system adversely. Often a patient will feel good initially when taking one of these medications but the feeling soon goes away. I have seen women who have tried every single antidepressant made and they still do not feel good. The doctors they have seen just keep prescribing different drugs and sometimes in combinations of as many as four prescriptions. So how, exactly, are these drugs working well?

Withdrawing From The Drugs

While some of these drugs are not classified as addictive, many of my patients report great difficulty in stopping them, saying, when they tried to stop, they feel worse than they did before they started taking the medication. Instead of being able to slowly reduce their dosage they've only been able to shave small pieces off the pills every few days in order to avoid terrible withdrawal side effects. Such difficulties have been especially true with SSRIs. Once off the medication, however, and past the withdrawal, these patients say they feel even better than they did while on the drug.

SSRIs and Children

Great Britain has banned the use of SSRI drugs for children and I hope that the United States will do the same. In 2002, *Patient Care* published a study in which the author initially described SSRIs as "relatively safe drugs." The American Academy of Child and Adolescent Psychiatry recommends SSRIs as the antidepressants of choice. Still the writer offered this caution, "Given the limited data on SSRI use in children and adolescents and the possibility of serious side effects, SSRIs may be used too often and psychotherapy not often enough." (Walsh, et al, 2002)

Cognitive Therapy, which focuses on the patient's present situation and coping options, can be very effective in helping depressive symptoms. One study found 75% of the cognitive therapy group was free of relapse while only 60 percent of those on medication could say the same. (Amsterdam, Archives of General Psychiatry)

Conversely, however, the text advocated the aggressive increase of dosages until children with major depressive disorders showed improvement and recommended SSRIs for obsessive compulsive disorder, social phobia, anxiety, eating disorders, autism, post-traumatic stress disorder, attention deficit disorder, and trichotillomania (hair pulling). Then there are statements regarding the side effects of overdosing and the claim that a psychiatric disorder can worsen from drugs. (Walsh, et al, 2002) And they call this science? The choice to play Russian roulette with our children's lives and our own lives should not be left to a doctor who doesn't even know the side effects of the drugs he prescribes.

Suicide in Adults Too

Do we think that only children and young adults kill themselves while taking SSRI drugs? Unfortunately that is not my experience. I know several adults who committed suicide while taking or coming off of these drugs. My cousin killed himself shortly after being prescribed Zoloft, my good friend's husband shot himself after stopping an antidepressant abruptly and a college friend killed himself on Prozac.

Bipolar, Psychiatric Label D'Jour

Although once a rare diagnosis, more and more patients come to me now labeled as "bipolar." One of the more dramatic cases involved James, a young man diagnosed while in high school. His symptoms began after a rough semester when he was not able to get enough sleep. Several nights each week he would study until 3 or 4 o'clock in the morning.

Sleep deprivation is known to cause serious psychological symptoms, but the psychiatrist James saw did not question him about his lifestyle. After listening to his symptoms, the doctor gave James the prescription drugs, Abilify and Lamictal. The drugs caused James to have difficulty swallowing. He experienced vomiting and gagging and then developed a rash. At this point the doctor switched James to Depakote, which also made him sick, so it was on to Zyprexa.

On Zyprexa, James started to drool and was so sleepy he began to have trouble in school. An honors student, James complained that his medication was effecting his education. The doctor added Neurontin, after which James became so depressed the doctor gave him Wellbutrin. This drug caused James to be anxious, so he then received Buspar. When the doctor slowly stopped the Zyprexa, James experienced fits of anger and self-destructive episodes.

The once popular young man began to isolate himself and on several occasions cut his wrists. Fearful for his own life, James asked to be placed in a psychiatric hospital. There he was verbally abused and threatened with restraint and heavy sedation if he did not do exactly as he was told. Thankfully, he was able to get out of the hospital before anything happened to him.

When James came to see me I took a complete history, performed a physical with lab work, and conducted allergy testing. I found James to have low blood sugar, allergies, and nutritional deficiencies. As we began to regulate his diet, restricting sweets and insuring adequate protein, James began to feel his depression and anxiety lift. James faced a lengthy process of being weaned off the many psychiatric drugs he was given, but his prognosis is good. I recently spoke to James and he informed me that he was now off all three psychiatric drugs. He came off of them slowly and felt much better each time he was able to stop one of the drugs. He says he is eating and sleeping well and feels like his old self again. He occasionally gets a feeling of anxiety but only if he does not eat right. Had the original physician, the psychiatrist, ordered similar medical testing or investigated James' sleep deprivation, so much of the boy's heartache could have been avoided.

Conclusion

In Appendix I, I have listed what I regard to be the complete protocol for a thorough evaluation as well as information on resources you as a patient may consult to educate yourself. In Appendix II, I have listed the possible cardiac and neurological side effects that can be caused from the many drugs that are prescribed for depression. I believe that no one should be prescribed an antidepressant without all of these issues being considered. With a thorough history and physical exam and lab work it is most likely that the underlying causes of a set of symptoms will be found and can be treated without resorting to antidepressants. Appendix III contains definitions of medical terms.

Remember, the Diagnostic and Statistical Manual states that all general medical conditions must be ruled out before a psychiatric diagnosis is made. Everyone deserves to have a physician who will take a thorough history, perform a complete physical exam, and be prepared to do as much lab work as needed to get to the bottom of a problem. In addition patients deserve informed consent -- full information on the potential side effects of a recommended treatment.

If all of this is done, I believe that most doctors will find, as I have, that the symptoms that previously were thought to be psychiatric in nature were, in fact, medical and could be successfully treated without psychiatric drugs. I believe that they will also conclude that depression is a symptom, not a disease and "Just Because You're Depressed, Doesn't Mean You Have Depression."

Appendix I
Protocol and Resources
or
Find the Cause and Fix the Problem

My Protocol for Diagnosing and Treating
The Underlying Causes of Depressed Symptoms

First consider if you are feeling depressed because of the loss of a loved one, pet or even something like your job. It is completely appropriate to be sad about these things. A two-week time period to get over such an experience is ridiculous. It takes as long as it takes. If you feel depressed and do not feel you have a reason for these feelings, consider the following plan. Find a doctor who will work with you to find the cause and fix the problem.

A Thorough History

A thorough history should be taken, including when the symptoms started and what was going on in the person's life at the time. It is also important to ask questions about the health of all body systems. If someone is constipated it may mean they are low in magnesium. If their hair is falling out, they may be hypothyroid.

A Complete Physical Exam

A complete physical exam should be performed. This includes blood pressure, temperature, heart rate, listening to the heart and lungs, examining the ears, nose and throat and checking the nervous system, including the reflexes.

Lab Tests

Complete Blood Count (Regular Lab) - Anemia can cause someone to feel depressed.

Fasting Metabolic Panel with electrolytes, liver function, blood glucose, cholesterol, triglycerides (Regular Lab) - Any abnormality here may indicate an underlying medical condition that can cause depressed feelings. High blood glucose indicates diabetes, high cholesterol may indicate low hormones or low thyroid, high triglycerides can indicate a problem metabolizing carbohydrates).

Thyroid Function: Total T3, Total T4, Free T3, Free T4, TSH, Thyroid Peroxidase Antibody, Thyroglobulin Antibody (Regular Lab) - The TSH can be done alone, but if it is normal, the rest of the tests must be performed along with the Basal Body Temperature or the Iodine Patch Test.

How to Take Basal Temperature: Shake down a glass thermometer the night before and place within reach of the bed. In the morning you do not move except to place the thermometer under your arm. Leave it there for ten minutes. Do not move. After ten minutes, remove and note the temperature. Do this for two mornings. If the temperature is greater than 97.8, repeat the procedure on the first and second days of your menstrual cycle. If temperatures are below 97.8 there is a possibility that you have hypothyroidism even if your lab work is normal.

Iodine Patch Test: Purchase a bottle of iodine at the drug store. Paint a 1-inch patch of iodine on the inner thigh and wait to see how quickly it absorbs or disappears. The iodine should last 24 hours. If it does not, you may be low in iodine and need to supplement it. Low iodine may be an indicator for hypothyroidism.

Nutritional Levels: White blood cell or red blood cell. - Some of these can be performed by a conventional laboratory but others will need a specialty lab that knows how to check for these nutritional deficiencies. White Blood Cell (SpectraCell), Red Blood Cell (Doctor's Data)

Magnesium Challenge Test (Regular Lab) – Even if the above nutritional tests are normal, the magnesium challenge should be performed. The patient collects urine for 24 hours, receives one or two injections of magnesium sulfate, 50% solution, depending on body weight, and collects urine for another 24 hours. To determine if the patient is low in magnesium, the following computation is performed:

> Amount of magnesium in 1st 24 hour urine sample
> xx mg
> Add amount of magnesium injected in 2 shots
> <u>200mg</u>
> Total magnesium available for excretion
> xxx mg
> Subtract amount of magnesium in 2nd 24 hour urine
> <u>xx mg</u>
> Amount of magnesium retained
> xxx mg
> Divide by 200 (amount of magnesium injected)
> xx = % retention

Any amount over 20% is considered low magnesium.

24 Hour Adrenal Test with Metabolites (Genova Diagnostics Labs.)

Hormone Tests: Blood Test if menopausal or taking hormones. - Pregnenalone, Progesterone, DHEA-S, Testosterone, Estradiol, Total Estrogen, (Conventional Lab) Hormone Saliva Test if not taking hormones or not menopausal: Should be 30 day saliva test and not a one time saliva test. It should check for estrogen, progesterone, DHEA and testosterone. (Diagnos-Techs)

Genetic Test for predisposition to certain medical and neurotransmitter problems and predisposition to problems metabolizing medications (Genova Diagnostics Lab)

Comprehensive Digestive Stool Analysis: This test should identify if too much yeast or pathogenic bacteria or parasites are in your intestinal tract. (Doctor's Data Lab)

Action in Response to Testing

Treat whatever lab abnormalities are found.

Allergy Testing to Foods and Inhalants

Be sure to _not_ take antihistamines or Vitamin C for one week before the allergy testing. Many antidepressants will interfere with the accuracy of allergy testing. It may be necessary to slowly and safely discontinue the antidepressants before allergy testing. Since tricyclic antidepressants are formulated from antihistamines, they will definitely interfere. SSRI's will not prevent a skin reaction from occurring during allergy testing but can interfere with observed reactions. I test allergies one at a time. This is the only way to determine which allergen could be causing the specific symptom for depression. Any psychotropic drug can interfere with allergy responses.

Test for Hypoglycemia

Change your diet. For breakfast, eat only protein and drink only water or black coffee. Eat protein snacks mid-morning, mid-afternoon and before bed. Eat protein with lunch and dinner. Remove all sweets from your diet and do not substitute artificial sweeteners, including aspartame (Nutrisweet and Equal) or sucralose (Splenda). Stevia is an herb that is very sweet and can be used as it does not affect blood sugar and is not synthetic.

Eat only protein, vegetables, no more than 2 fruits/day and

whole grains. If you feel better with this eating plan, continue on it, as Hypoglycemia is the likely cause of your symptoms.

Exercise

A study conducted by the Public Health Institute in Berkeley, California examined the effect of exercise on depression. They used an 8-point scale to rate the amount of physical activity performed. For every one point increase in physical activity, there was a 10% decrease in the risk of being depressed and a 17% decrease in the risk of becoming depressed. I tend to think that walking is the best exercise as almost anyone can do it and you are less likely to hurt yourself. I recommend to my patients that they walk 30 minutes a day at least 4 times each week.

Try Acupuncture

It also might help your mood. After 8 weeks of acupuncture, a group of women with major depression symptoms reported results similar to taking antidepressants according to University of Arizona researchers.

Just Because You're Depressed

Recommended Reading:

Books by John Lee, MD
What Your Doctor May Not Tell You About Breast Cancer,
Warner Books, *2005*
What Your Doctor May Not Tell You About Menopause,
Warner Books, 2004
What Your Doctor May Not Tell You About Pre-Menopause,
Warner Books, 2005

Hypothyroidism, The Unsuspected Illness by Broda Barnes, MD,
Harper & Row, 1976

Prozac, Panacea or Pandora by Ann Tracy, PhD, Cassia
Publications, 1994

Books by David Brownstein, MD
Iodine: Why You Need It, Why You Can't Live Without It,
Medical Alternative Press, 2004
Overcoming Thyroid Disorders, Medical Alternative Press,
2002
Salt: Your Way To Health, Medical Alternative Press, 2005
The Guide to Healthy Eating, Medical Alternative Press,
2005
Overcoming Arthritis, Medical Alternative Press, 2000

Safe Uses of Cortisone by William Jefferies, MD, C.C. Thomas,
Springfield, Ill.,1996

Fight for Your Health, Exposing the FDA's Betrayal of America
by Byron J. Richards, Wellness Resources Books (2006)

The Myth of Osteoporosis by Gillian Sanson, MCD Century
Publications, 2003

Books by Thomas Szasz, MD
The Myth of Mental Illness, HarperCollins Publishers,
1974
The Manufacture of Madness, Syracuse Publishing, 1997

Books by Mary Ann Block, DO
    No More ADHD, Block Books, 2001
    No More Antibiotics, Kensington Publishing, 1998
    Today I Will Not Die, Kensington Publishing, 2001
    The ABC's of Raising Great Kids. Block Publishing, 2005
    No More Ritalin, Kensington Publishing, 1996

Web Sites:

Drugawareness.org
CCHR.org
alternativementalhealth.org
wellnessresources.com
blockcenter.com
ssristories.com

Appendix II

The following is a list of some of the antidepressants and other drugs often prescribed for depression and some of the side effects listed by the manufacturer I have only listed the cardiac and nervous system side effects listed in the PDR. There are many other side effects reported.

I tell my patients to read the side effects reported by the drug companies. If they do not want to live with one of the side effects, they should look for another treatment. The patient, not the doctor, should decide if the benefit of the drug is worth the risk. The doctor will not have to live with the side effect. The patient will. The only way to make good, educated decisions about your treatments is to know what your options are and the risks of those options.

Definitions of medical terms follow.

Every drug listed, except the benzodiazepines, have a potentially fatal side effect such as myocardial infarction (heart attack), sudden death, cardiac arrest or heart failure. However, I was taught in medical school that "cold turkey" withdrawal from benzodiazepines could be fatal.

SSRI's
Prozac and Seraphem (fluoxetine hydrochloride)

Cardiovascular System
Hemorrhage, hypertension, angina pectoris, arrhythmia, congestive **heart failure**, hypotension, migraine, **myocardial infarction**, postural hypotension, syncope, tachycardia, vascular headache, atrial fibrillation, bradycardia, cerebral embolism, cerebral ischemia, cerebrovascular accident, extrasystoles, heart arrest, heart block, pallor, peripheral vascular disorder, phlebitis, shock, thrombophlebitis, thrombosis, vasospasm, ventricular arrhyia, ventricular extrasystoles, ventricular fibrillation

Nervous System

Agitation, amnesia, confusion, emotional liability, sleep disorder, abnormal gait, acute brain syndrome, akathisia, apathy, ataxia, buccoglossal syndrome, CNS depression, CNS stimulation, depersonalization, euphoria, hallucinations, hostility, hyperkinesia, hypertonia, hypesthesia, incoordination, libido increased, myoclonus, neuralgia, neuropathy, neurosis, paranoid reactions, personality disorder, psychosis, vertigo, abnormal electroencephalogram, antisocial reaction, circumoral paresthesia, coma, delusions, dysarthria, dystonia, extrapyramidal syndrome, foot drop, hyperesthesia, neuritis, paralysis, reflexes decreased, stupor

Paxil (paroxetine hydrochloride)

Cardiovascular System

Hypertension, tachycardia, bradycardia, hematoma, hypotension, migraine, syncope, angina pectoris, arrhythmia nodal, atrial fibrillation, bundle branch block, cerebral ischemia, cerebrovascular accident, congestive heart failure, heart block, low cardiac output, **myocardial infarction**, myocardial ischemia, pallor, phlebitis, pulmonary embolus, supraventricular, extrasystoles, thrombophlebitis, thrombosis, varicose vein, vascular headache, ventricular extrasystoles

Nervous System

Emotional liability, vertigo, abnormal thinking, alcohol abuse, ataxia, delirium, dystonia, dyskinesia, euphoria, hallucinations, hostility, hypertonia, hypesthesia, hypokinesia, incoordination, lack of emotion, libido increased, manic reaction, neurosis, paralysis, paranoid reaction, psychosis, abnormal gait, akinesia, antisocial reaction, aphasia, choreoathetosis, circumoral paresthesias, convulsion, delusions, diplopia, drug dependence, dysarthria, extrapyramidal syndrome, fasciculations, grand mal convulsion, hyperalgesia, hysteria, manic-depressive reaction, meningitis, myelitis, neuralgia, neuropathy, nystagmus, peripheral neuritis, psychotic depression, reflexes decreased, reflexes increased, stupor, torticollis, trimus, withdrawal syndrome

Luvox (Fluvoxamine Maleate)

Cardiovascular System
Hypertension, hypotension, syncope, tachycardia, angina pectoris, bradycardia, cardiomyopathy, cardiovascular disease, cold extremities, conduction delay, heart failure, **myocardial infarction**, pallor, pulse irregular, ST segment changes, AV block, cerebrovascular accident, coronary artery disease, embolus, pericarditis, phlebitis, pulmonary infarction, supraventricular extrasystoles

Nervous System
Amnesia, apathy, hyperkinesia, hypokinesia, manic reaction, myoclonus, psychotic reaction, agoraphobia, akathisia, ataxia, CNS depression, convulsion, delirium, delusion, depersonalization, drug dependence, dyskinesia, dystonia, emotional lability, euphoria, extrapyramidal syndrome, gait unsteady, hallucinations, hemiplegia, hostility, hypersomnia, hypochondriasis, hypotonia, hysteria, incoordination, increased salivation, increased libido, neuralgia, paralysis, paranoid reaction, phobia, psychosis, sleep disorder, stupor, twitching, vertigo, akinesia, coma, fibrillations, mutism, obsessions, reflexes decreased, slurred speech, tardive dyskinesia, torticollis, trismus, withdrawal syndrome.

Zoloft (sertraline hydrochloride)

Cardiovascular System
Palpitations, chest pain, hypertension, tachycardia, postural dizziness, postural hypotension, periorbitaledema, peripheral edema, hypotension, peripheal ischemia, syncope, edema, dependent edema, precordial chest pain, substernal chest pain, aggravated hypertension, **myocardial infarction**, cerebrovascular disorder.

Nervous System
Hypertonia, hypoesthesia, twitching, confusion,

hyperkinesia, vertigo, ataxia, migraine, abnormal coordination, hyperesthesia, leg cramps, abnormal gait, nystagmus, hypokinesia, dysphonia, coma, dyskinesia, hypotonia, ptosis, choreathetosis, hyporefelxia.

Celexa (citalopram hydrobromide)

Cardiovascular System:
Tachycardia, postural hypotension, hypertension, bradycardia, edema, angina pectoris, extrasystoles, heart failure, flushing, **myocardial infarction**, cerebrovascular accident, myocardial ischemia, transient ischemia attack, phlebitis, atrial fibrillation, cardiac arrest, bundle branch block

Central and Peripheral Nervous System
Paresthesia, migraine, hyperkinesia, vertigo, hypertonia, extrapyramidal disorder, leg cramps, involuntary muscle contractions, hypokinesia, ataxia, abnormal coordination, hyperesthesia, ptosis, stupor

Serotonin and Norepinephrine Reuptake Inhibitors

Effexor (venlafaxine hydrochloride)

Cardiovascular System
Migraine, angina pectoris, arrhythmia, extrasystoles, hypotension, peripheral pectoris, vascular disorder, syncope, thrombophlebitis, arteritis, first-degree artrioventricular block, bigeminy, bradycardia, bundle branch block, cerebral ischemia, coronary artery disease, congestive heart failure, **heart arrest**, mitral valve disorder, mucocutaneous hemorrhage, **myocardial infarction**, pallor

Nervous System
Emotional lability, trismus, vertigo, apathy, ataxia, circumoral parethesia, CNS stimulation, euphoria, halluncinations, hostility, hyperesthesia, hyperkinesia, hypotonia, incoordination, libido increased, manic reaction,

myoclonus, neuralgia, neuropathy, paranoid reaction, psychosis, seizure, abnormal speech, stupor, akathisia, akinesia, alcohol abuse, aphasia, bradykinesia, buccoglossal syndrome, cerebrovascular accident, loss of consciousness, delusions, dementia, dystonia, facial paralysis, abnormal gait, Guillain-Barre Syndrome, hypokinesia, neuritis, nystagmus, psychotic depression, reflexes decreased, reflexes increased, suicidal ideation, torticollis

Serzone (nefazodone hydrochloride)

Cardiovascular System
Tachycardia, hypertension, synope, ventricular extrasystoles, and angina pectoris, AV block, congestive **heart failure,** hemorrhage, pallor, and varicose vein.

Nervous System
Vertigo, twitching, depersonalization, hallucinations, suicide attempt, apathy, euphoria, hostility, suicidal thoughts, abnormal gait, thinking abnormal, attention decreased, derealization, neuralgia, paranoid reaction, dysarthria, increased libido, suicide and myoclonus, hyperkinesia, increased salivation, cerebrovascular accident, hyperesthesia, hypotonia, ptosis, and neuroleptic malignant syndrome.

Selective Serotonin and Norepinephrine Reuptake Inhibitor

Cymbalta

Cardiovascular System
Palpitations, atrial fibrillation, **myocardial infarction,** tachycardia, coronary artery disease, cardiac failure, **congestive cardiac failure,** EKG changes, hypertensive crisis, supraventricualr arrhythmia, hypotension

Nervous System
Lethargy, parasthesia, abnormal coordination, dyskinesia, hypersomnia, myoclonus, dysarthria, extrapyramidal disorder, hallucinations, agitation,

anxiety, decreased libido, nightmares, apathy, irritability, confused state, mood swings, suicide, mania

Norepinephrine and Dopamine Reuptake Inhibitors

WellButrin (bupropion hydrochloride)

Cardiovascular System
Hypertension, orthostatic hypotension, third degree heart block, tachycardia, stroke, **myocardial infarction**, pulmonary embolism

Nervous System
Coma, delirium, dream abnormalities, paresthesia, unmasking of tardive duskinesia

Benzodiazepines

Valium, Ativan, Librium, Xanax, Klonopin, Serax, Tranxene, Dalmane, Doral, Restoril

Cardiovascular System
Minor changes in EEG patterns, usually low-voltage fast activity, have been observed in patients during and after Valium therapy, chest pain, postural hypotension, palpitations

Nervous System
Drowsiness, fatigue, and ataxia. Infrequently encountered were confusion, constipation, depression, diplopia, dysarthria, headache, hypotension, incontinence, jaundice, changes in libido, nausea, changes in salivation, skin rash, slurred speech, tremor, urinary retention, worsening of seizures, vertigo and blurred vision, paradoxical reactions such as acute hyperexcited states, anxiety, hallucinations, increased muscle spasticity, insomnia, rage, sleep disturbances and stimulation.

Tricyclic Antidepressants

Tofranil (imipramine hydrochloride), Norpramin, Anafranil, Elavil, Pamelor, Sinequan, Surmontil

Cardiovascular System
Dysrhythmias, orthostatic hypotension, hypertension, syncope, tachycardia, palpitations, **myocardial infarction**, arrhythmias, heart block, precipitation of CHF, stroke

Nervous System
Dry mouth, blurred vision, disturbance of accommodations for near visions, mydriasis, increased intraocular pressure, confusion, disturbed concentration, hallucinations, disorientation, decreased memory, feelings of reality, delusions, anxiety, nervousness, restlessness, agitation, panic, insomnia, nightares, hypomania, mania, exacerbation of psychosis, drowsiness, weakness, fatigue, headache, numbness, tingling, paresthesias of extremities, incoordination, motor hyperactivity, akathisia, ataxia, tremors, peripheral neuropthy, extrapyramidal symptoms, seizures, speech blockage, dysarthria, tinnitus, altered EEG

Norpramin has a Black Box Warning saying it can cause sudden cardiac death in children. It also says it is not indicated for children. In spite of that, Shana Dunkel's psychiatrist prescribed it to her in doses that exceeded recommendations for adolescents. Shana died in her mother's arms.

Other
Risperdal (resperidone)

Cardiovascular System
Hypertension, **myocardial infarction**, angina pectoris, palpitations, AV block,   premature atrial contractions, EKG abnormalities, pulmonary embolism myocarditis, atrial

fibrillation, **sudden death, cardiopulmonary arrest**

Nervous System
Double vision, tardive dyskinesia, seizures, cognitive and motor impairment, suicide, headache, dizziness, diminished sexual desire, depression, catatonic reaction, emotional lability, delirium, stupor, tongue paralysis, coma, migraine

Risperdal has also been shown to cause diabetes

Remeron (mirtazapine)

Cardiovascular System
Hypertension, vasodilation, angina pectoris, bradycardia, ventricular extrasystoles, **myocardial infarction,**syncope, migraine, hypotension, atrial arrhythmia, bigeminy, vascular headache, pulmonary embolus, cerebral ischemia, cardiomegaly, phlebitis, left heart failure

Nervous System
Hypethesia, apathy, depression, hypokinesia, vertigo, twitching, agitation, anxiety, amnesia, hyperkinesia, paresthesia, ataxia, delirium, delusions, depersonalization, dypkinesia, extrapyramidal syndrome, libido increased, coordination abnormal, dysarthria, hallucinations, manic reaction, neurosis, dystonia, hostility, reflexes increased, emotional liability, euphoria, paranoid reaction, aphasia, nystagmus, akathisia, stupor, dementia, diplopia, drug dependence, paralysis, grand mal convulsion, hypertonia, myoclonus, psychotic depression, withdrawal syndrome

Nardil (Phenelzine Sulfate Tablets, USP)

Cardiovascular System
Postural hypotension, edema, **fatal hypertensive crisis**

Nervous System
Dizziness, headache, drowsiness, sleep disturbances, (including insomnia and hypersomnia) fatigue, weakness, tremors, twitching, myoclonic movements, hyperreflexia,

Jitteriness, palilalia, euphoria, nystagmus, paresthesias, ataxia, shock-like coma, toxic delirium, manic reaction, convulsions, acute anxiety reaction, precipitation of schizophrenia, transient respiratory and cardiovascular depression following ECT.

Thioridazine Hydrochloride Tablets, USP

Cardiovascular System
ECG changes have been reported. Several sudden and unexpected deaths apparently due to **cardiac arrest** have occurred in patients previously showing characteristic electrocardiographic changes while taking the drug, hypotension.

Nervous System
Drowsiness, Pseudo-parkinsonism and other extrapyramidal symptoms, nocturnal confusion, hyperactivity, lethargy, psychotic reactions, restlessness, and headache have been reported but are extremely rare, dryness of mouth, blurred vision, constipation, nausea, vomiting, diarrhea, nasal stuffiness, and pallor.

Haldol

Cardiovascular System
Tachycardia, hypotension, hypertension, EKG changes, **sudden and unexpected death**.

Nervous System
Tardive dyskinesia, extrapyramidal symptoms, visual disturbances, blurred vision, cataracts.

Clozaril

Cardiovascular System
Orthostatic hypotension, tachycardia, EKG changes, ischemic changes, arrhythmias, **myocardial infarction, sudden death**, pulmonary embolism, diabetes, hepatitis,

chest pain,

Nervous System
Seizures, neuroleptic malignant syndrome, tardive
dyskinesia, mental and physical impairment, visual
disturbances,drowsiness, vertigo, headache, tremor,
restlessness, agitation, rigidity, akathisia, confusion, lethargy,
ataxia, slurred speech, depression, anxiety

Compazine

Cardiovascular System
EKG changes, **cardiac arrest**

Nervous System
Neuroleptic malignant syndrome, tardive dyskinesia, motor
restlessness, dystonia, Pseudo-parkinson's syndrome,
akathisia, seizures, brain swelling, catatonic

Stelazine

Cardiovascular System
EKG changes, **sudden death**, hypotension, **cardiac arrest**

Nervous System
Extrapyramidal reactions, Neuroleptic malignant syndrome,
dystonia, motor restlessness, Pseudo-parkinson's, tardive
dyskinesia, akathisia, seizures, brain swelling, catatonic
Trilafon

Cardiovascular System
Tachycardia, postural hypotension, bradycardia, **cardiac
arrest**, dizziness, **sudden death**

Nervous System
Extrapyramidal reactions, numbness, trismus, torticollis,
slurred speech, dysphagia, akathisia, parkinsonism, ataxia,
tardive dyskinesia, seizures, neuroleptic malignant
syndrome, catatonic state, paranoia, lethargy

Geodon

Cardiovascular System
Tachycardia, **sudden death**, postural hypotension, hypertension, bradycardia, angina pectoris, pulmonary embolus, stroke, myocarditis, EKG changes

Nervous System
Extrapyramidal reactions, seizures, akithesia, dystonia, dizziness, agitation, tremor, paresthesia, vertigo, delirium, akinesia, diplopia, trismus, neuropathy

Thorazine

Cardiovascular System
EKG changes, **sudden death**, hypotension, tachycardia

Nervous System
Extrapyramidal reactions, psychosis, catatonic, parkinsonism, tardive dyskinesia, seizures, catatonic state, paranoia, lethargy

Zyprexa

Cardiovascular System
Hypotension, bradycardia, congestive heart failure, **cardiac arrest**, heart palpitation, pulmonary embolism

Nervous System
Schizophrenia, amnesia, ataxia, antisocial, delirium, hypoesthesia, hypokinesia, phobias, dykinesia, stupor, vertigo, neuropathey, brain hemorrhage

Vistaril (hydroxyzine pamoate)

Cardiovascular System
Stroke, heart block, **myocardial infarction**, arrhythmias, hypotension, particularly orthostatic hypotension,

hypertension, tachycardia, palpitation.

Nervous System
Seizures, incoordination, ataxia, tremors, peripheral
neuropathy, numbness, tingling, and paresthesias of
extremities, weakness and fatigue, headache, syndrome of
inappropriate ADH secretion, tinnitus, alteration in EEG
patterns

Etrafon (perphenazine and amitriptyline hydrochloride)

Cardiovascular System
Postural hypotension, tachycardia, bradycardia, **cardiac
arrest**, faintness, and dizziness. Occasionally the
hypotensive effect may produce a shock-like condition. ECG
changes, nonspecific, usually reversible, have been observed
in some patients receiving phenothiazine

Nervous System
Extrapyramidal reactions, opisthotonus, trismus, torticollis,
retrocollis, aching and numbness of the limbs, motor
restlessness, oculogyric crisis, hyperreflexia, dystonia,
including protrusion, discoloration, aching and rounding of
the tongue, tonic spasm of the masticatory muscles, tight
feeling in the throat, slurred speech, dysphagia, akathisia,
dyskinesia, parkinsonism, and ataxia, cerebral edema,
abnormality of cerebrospinal fluid proteins, convulsive
seizures, particularly in patients with EEG abnormalities or a
history of such disorders, and headaches. Neuroleptic
malignant syndrome has been reported in patients treated
with neuroleptic drugs. Adverse behavioral effects include
paradoxical exacerbation of psychotic symptoms, catatonic-
like states, paranoid reactions, lethargy, paradoxical
excitement, restlessness, hyperactivity, nocturnal confusion,
bizarre dreams, and insomnia. Hyperreflexia has been
reported in the newborn when a phenothiazine was used
during pregnancy.

Vivactil (protriptyline HCL)

Cardiovascular System
Heart block, **myocardial infarction**, hypotension, tachycardia, hypertension, palpitations.

Nervous System
Seizures, ataxia, tremors, extrapyramidal symptoms, dizzy, headache, confusion, delusions, hallucinations, agitation, psychosis, panic, restlessness.

Depakote

Cardiovascular System
Tachycardia, hypertension, palpitations.
Life threatening pancreatitis, fatal liver damage

Nervous System
Ataxia, tremors, dizzy, amnesia, depression, blurred vision, headache, anxiety, confusion, personality disorder, hallucinations, vertigo, dementia.

Just Because You're Depressed

Appendix III
Definitions of Terms

Cardiovascular System Side Effects:

angina pectoris: chest pain due to lack of oxygen to the heart

arrhythmia: abnormal heart rhythm

atrial fibrillation: rapid: irregular heart contractions

bradycardia: slow heart rate

bundle branch block: impairment of heart function

cardiomyopathy: heart disease

cardiovascular disease: heart disease

conduction delay: slowing of energy of the heart

cerebral embolism: blocking of an artery to the brain

cerebral ischemia: blocking of blood to the brain

cerebrovascular accident: stroke

congestive heart failure: abnormal accumulation of blood in the heart

coronary artery disease: diseases of the arteries to the heart

extrasystole: premature heart contraction that is independent of the normal heart rhythm

embolus: artery blockage

heart arrest: stopping of heart function

heart block: impairment of heart function

heart failure: inability of the heart to meet the body's needs

hematoma: blood clot

hemorrhage: bleeding

hypertension: high blood pressure

hypotension: low blood pressure

low cardiac output: inadequate pumping of the blood from the heart

migraine: headaches associated with changes of the blood vessels in the brain

myocardial infarction: heart attack

myocardial ischemia: blocking of blood to the heart

opisthotonus: spasm in which the head and heels are bent backwards

pallor: pale

pericarditis: inflammation of the sac enclosing the heart

peripheral vascular disorder: blood vessel problems

phlebitis: inflammation of a vein

postural hypotension: low blood pressure when going from seated to standing

pulmonary embolus: blocking of an artery to the lungs

pulmonary infarction: death of lung tissue due to obstruction of blood flow

shock: circulation failure causing low blood pressure, coldness and rapid heart rate

syncope: loss of consciousness

tachycardia: rapid heart rate

thrombophlebitis: vein inflammation associated with a blood clot

thrombosis: blood clot

varicose veins: unnaturally and permanently distended vein

vascular headache: see migraine

vasospasm: blood vessel spasms

ventricular arrhythmia: irregular heart contractions

ventricular fibrillation: rapid, irregular heart contractions

Nervous System Side Effects:

abnormal electroencephalogram: changes in electrical potential of the brain

abnormal gait: abnormal walking

agoraphobia: severe dread of open spaces

akathisia: anxiety: restlessness

akinesia: absence of movements

amnesia: loss of memory

antisocial reaction: repeated conflict with society

apathy: lack of feelings or emotions

aphasia: inability to communicate

ataxia: irregularity of muscle actions

choreoathetosis: rapid, jerky, involuntary motions

CNS depression: flattened or below normal level function of the nervous system

CNS stimulation: excited or above normal level function of the nervous system

coma: unconsciousness

confusion: disturbed orientation

convulsion: involuntary contractions of the muscles

delirium: having illusions, delusions, hallucinations, incoherence, restlessness

delusions: a false personal belief maintained in spite of proof to the contrary

depersonalization: loss of self perception and change of reality

diplopia: double vision

dysarthria: speech disturbance

dyskinesia: movement impairment

dystonia: muscle impairment

emotional lability: emotionally unstable

euphoria: abnormal or exaggerated sense of well-being

extrapyramidal syndrome: abnormal, involuntary movements

fasciculations: abnormal muscle contractions seen under the skin

foot drop: foot hangs due to nerve damage

grand mal convulsion: seizure

hallucinations: abnormal sense of perception

hemiplegia: paralysis of one side of the body

hypochondriasis: morbid anxiety about one's health

hypotonia: decreased muscle tone

hyperalgesia: diminished sense of pain

hyperesthesia: increased sensitivity to stimulation

hyperkinesias: abnormally increased motor activity

hypersomnia: excessive sleep or drowsiness

hypertonia: increased tone of muscles

hypesthesia: abnormally decreased sensitivity to stimulation

hypokinesia: abnormally diminished motor activity

hysteria: lack of control over emotions

incoordination: lack of control of muscle actions

libido increased: increased sexual desire

manic reaction: extreme excitement

manic-depressive reaction: alternating between extreme excitement and depression

meningitis: inflammation of the brain membranes

mutism: unable to speak

myelitis: spinal cord inflammation

myoclonus: shock-like contractions of the muscles

neuralgia: nerve pain

neuritis: nerve inflammation

neuropathy: any disturbance of the nervous system

neurosis: hysterical symptoms of anxiety, panic and unjustified dread

nystagmus: involuntary movements of the eyeball

obsessions: persistent unwanted impulses that can't be eliminated with reason

paralysis: loss of motor or sensory function

paranoid reactions: delusions of grandeur and persecution

phobia: abnormal fear

psychosis: derangement of personality and loss of contact with reality

reflexes decreased: decreased nervous system response

reflexes increased: increased nervous system response

stupor: reduced responsiveness

tardive dyskinesia: irreversible, involuntary movements

trismus: spasm of muscles affecting the ability of opening the jaw

torticollis: contracted neck muscles

vertigo: feeling that self is moving or that surroundings are moving

withdrawal syndrome: retreat from reality

WORKS CITED

American Journal of Clinical Nutrition 1971: 24:432-43.
American Journal of Psychiatry 2006, Sep.: 163(9): 1519-30
American Psychiatric Association: Diagnostic and Statistical
    Manual of Mental Disorders 4th Edition, Text Revision.
    Washington, DC. 2000.
Amsterdam Jay D., et al. "Cognitive Therapy as Good as
    Antidepressants, Effects Last Longer." Archives of General
    Psychiatry
Archives of Internal Medicine. "Depression in Association with
    Severe Obesity." 2003: p. 163:2058-2065.
Argyropoulos, S.V., Hood, S.D., Adrover, M., Bell, C.J., Rich, A.S.,
    Nash, J.R., Rich, N.C., Witchel, H.J., Nutt, D.J. "Tryptophan
    depletion reverses the therapeutic effect of selective
    serotonin reuptake inhibitors in social anxiety disorder."
    Biological Psychiatry 2004, Oct 1: 56 (7):503-9.
Associated Press. "Doctor apologizes for obscuring financial
    ties." Washington Post June 30, 2002.

Barnes, B. & Galton, L. Hypothyroidism, The Unsuspected
    Illness New York: Ty Crowell Co., 1976.
Barrett, G. "Depression in Kids, Antidepressant: Are They
    Needed For Children?" Chillicothe Gazette 2004, March 14.
Bell, I.R., Jasnoski, M.L., Kagan, J, King, D.S. "Depression and
    allergies: survey of a non-clinical population". Psychother
    Psychosom 1991: 55(1):24-31.
Block, Mary Ann. No More ADHD. Block Books, 2001.
Borok, G., et al, "Atopy: The Incidence in Chronic Recurrent
    Maladies," XVI European Congress of Allergy and Clinical
    Immunology, June 24-25, 1995, British Journal of Child
    Psychology and Psychiatry
British Medical College of Psychiatry 2003: p. 3:17
British Medical College of Psychiatry 2005, 19 Feb.: p. 330:396
Brooks, K., "Yates gets life in prison." Fort Worth Star-Telegram
    2002, March 16: 1A
Brown, D., Gaby, A.R. & Reichert, R. "Altering the Brain's
    Chemistry to Elevate Mood." Nutrition Science News 1999,
    Feb.

Brown, D., Gaby, A.R. & Reichert, R. "Natural Remedies for Depression." Nutrition Science News 1999, Feb.

Brownstein, D., Iodine: Why You Need It, Why You Can't Live Without It. Published by David Brownstein, M.D., 5821 W. Maple Rd, Suite 192, West Bloomfield, MI 48322

Brownstein, D., Overcoming Thyroid Disorders. Published by David Brownstein, M.D., 5821 W. Maple Rd, Suite 192, West Bloomfield, MI 48322

Cato, J. "Pitan tragedy detailed in letter, Anti-depressant dosage increased days before killings." The Herald Rock Hill, SC. 2004, Feb.

Chaker, A.M. "Shop till you stop, with the help of medication." Fort Worth Star-Telegram. 2003, Jan 4: 5F

Citizens Commission on Human Rights. "Psychiatrists Advised FDA 17 Years Ago Not to Act on Suicide and Homicidal Antidepressant Risks." 2004, Sept. 9.

Citizens Commission on Human Rights 2005. Direct link: www.cchr.org/fraud/eng/page 29 a.h.

Citizens Commission on Human Rights 2004. Antidepressants and Suicide. Texas.

Cosgrove, Lisa, et al, Financial Ties between DSM-IV Panel Members and the Pharmaceutical Industry. 2006: 75:154-160

Cotterchio, M., et al, "Antidepressant Medication Use and Breast Cancer Risk." American Journal of Epidemiology 2000: p.151:951-57

Davidson, J., Sjoerdsma, A., Loomis, L.N., Udenfriend, S., "Studies with the serotonin precursor, 5-hydroxytryptophan, in experimental animals and man." Journal of Clinical Investigation. 1957. Nov. 36(11):1594-9.

Dorland's Medical Dictionary, 23rd Edition

Facchinetti, F., et al. "Oral magnesium successfully relieves premenstrual mood changes." Obstet Gynecol 78: 1991, p. 177-181.

FDA Public Health Advisory, Reports of Suicidality in Pediatrics Oct 27, 2003.

Fecher, L. "Review of Medical Records, Andrea Yates" Medical Director of Citizens Commission on Human Rights. 2002, Mar. 4.

Flynn, Paul. Hot News Feb 24, 2004.

Frizel, D., et al. "Plasma, magnesium, and calcium in depression." British Journal of Psychiatry. 1969 Vol. 115 (529):1375-1377.

Graedon, J. & T., "Big Pharma's little secret." Fort Worth Star-Telegram Jan. 19, 2004.

Graedon, J. & T., "Drug ad rules easing further." Fort Worth Star-Telegram February 23, 2004.

Gregg, Valerie. Burden of Proof. Spring, 2003.

Gregory, T. "Understanding Depression in Women." Patient Care 1999, Nov. 30: p. 28

Guyton, Arthur. Textbook of Medical Physiology, Eighth edition. WB Saunders Co. 1991: p. 371

Hogan, B. "Pulling Strings From Afar." AARP Bulletin. 2003, Feb.: p. 4

Home News Tribune "FDA: 157 Million Prescriptions for Newer Antidepressants." Mar 8, 2004.

Huppke "Lily Moving On After Losing Prozac Patent Appeal" AP 2001. Indianapolis

James, G. "Advances in Depression Treatment: Better Mental Health and Longer Lives for Your Patients." Osteopathic Family Physician News. 2002, June/July: p. 20.

Jarvis, J. "Trial puts focus on insanity defense." Fort Worth Star-Telegram. 2002, Mar. 11: 1A

Jefferies, W. Safe Uses of Cortisone. C.C. Thomas, Springfield, Ill. 1996

Kohn, L.T., Corrigan, J.M. & Donaldson, M.S., editors. To Err Is Human: Building A Safer Health System, National Academies Press, 2000.

Lazarou, J., et al. "Incidence of Adverse Drug Reactions in Hospitalized Patients." Journal of the American Medical Association. 1998, Apr. 15: Vol. 279: p. 1200-1205.

Lee, J. & Hopkins, V. <u>What Your Doctor May Not Tell You About Menopause.</u> New York: Warner Books, Jan. 2002.

Lee, J. <u>What Your Doctor May Not Tell You About Women's Breast Cancer.</u> Recorded Books, 2002.

Lishman, W.A. <u>Organic Psychiatry, The Psychological Consequences of Cerebral Disease.</u> Third Edition, Blackwell Publishing Company, 1978.

Marshall, P.S., et al. "Effects of seasonal allergic rhinitis on fatigue levels and mood." <u>Psychosom Med.</u> 2002, Jul/Aug: 64:684-9.

Mathews, A.W. "FDA Revisits Issue of Antidepressants for Youths, New Analysis May Pressure Agency to Set Limit on Use Because of Suicide Risk." <u>Wall Street Journal</u> 2004, Aug. 5: A1

Morgan K.J., et al. "Magnesium and calcium dietary intakes of the U.S. population." <u>Journal American College of Nutrition</u> 1985: Vol. 4:195-206

Morris, M. <u>Psychotherapy and Psychosomatics</u> 2003, March/April edition: p. 72, 2:80-7

Nasr, S., et al, <u>Concordance of atopic and affective disorders, J. Affective Disorders.</u> 1981. 3:291

Neergaard, L. "Vaccine tests aim to fight lethal diarrhea." <u>Fort Worth Star-Telegram</u> 2002, Jul 9: 3A

Neergaard, L. "Feds Say Doctors Don't Head Drug Warnings." <u>Associated Press</u> 2000, Dec 12.

O'Meara, K.P. "Parents Plead for Lives of Children." <u>Insightmag.com.</u> 2004, Mar. 24.

Ossofsky, H.J. "Affective and atopic disorders and cyclic AMP." <u>Compr Psychiatry</u> 1976: 17:335

Patterson, K. "Antidepressants endorsed for teens." <u>Dallas Morning News</u> 2004, Jan. 22: 1A

Pear, R. "In a Shift, Bush Moves to Block Medical Suits." <u>New York Times</u> 2004, July 25.

Phillips, J. " Dear Abby." <u>Fort Worth Star-Telegram</u> 2003, July 5: 2F

Phillips, J. " Dear Abby." Fort Worth Star-Telegram 2001, Nov.26: 4D

Physician's Desk Reference 2006

Polk, J. "Teen Gets 30 Years in Zoloft Case." CNN 2005, Feb. 16.

Praschak-Rieder, N., Hussey, D., Wilson, A.A., Carella, A., Lee, M., Dunn, E., Willeit, M., Bagby, R.M., Houle, S., Meyer, J.H. " Tryptophan depletion and serotonin loss in selective serotonin reuptake inhibitor-treated depression." Biological Psychiatry. 2004, Oct 15: 56(8):587-91.

Pugh, T. "Onslaught of drug ads overwhelms FDA." Fort Worth Star-Telegram. 2004, Feb. 1: 1F

Richards, Byron J. Fight for Your Health, Exposing the FDA's Betrayal of America. Wellness Resources Books. 2006

Richardson, E. "Pharmacology of antidepressants in use in the United States." Journal of Clinical Psychiatry 1982: 43:4

Rippere, V. "Some varieties of food intolerance in psychiatric patients: An overview." Nutr. Health 3, 1984 (3):125-36,

Sanders, A.& Colliver, V. "Antidepressants Hazardous to Health Care Coverage, Insurance Plans Stymie Individual Policyholders." San Francisco Chronicle Feb. 22, 2004.

Sanson, G. The Myth of Osteoporosis: What Every Woman Should Know About Creating Bone Health. MCD Century Publications, Ann Arbor, MI 48105, 2003.

Singh, A., et al. "Magnesium, zinc, and copper status of US Navy SEAL trainees." American Journal of Clinical Nutrition 1989: p.49:695-700

Smart Publications "How Can We Trust Research Studies When Scientists Often Have a Conflict of Interest?" Petaluma, CA. 2004, Direct Link: www.smart-publications.com/articles/ 040126researchstudies.h

Springer, J. " Prosecutor: 'Evil' Boy Planned Gruesome Murder Of His Grandparents." Court TV. 2005, Feb. 1.

Starfield, B. "Medical Errors – A Leading Cause of Death." Journal of American Medical Association. 284, No.4.

Sugerman, A.A., Southern, D.L., Curran, J.F. "A study of antibody levels in alcoholic, depressive and schizophrenic patients." Ann Allergy 1982: 48(3):166-171.

Szasz, T. S. <u>Myth of Mental Illness: Foundations of a Theory of Personal Conduct</u>. New York: HarperCollins, 1974.

Temple, R. and Himmel, M. "Safety of Newly Approved Drugs." <u>Journal of the American Medical Association</u> 2002, May 1: 287:2273-2275s

Udenfriend, Sidney, Herbert Weissbach, and Donald F. Bogdanski, "Increase in tissue serotonin following administration of its precursor 5-hydroxytryptophan." Journal of Biological Chemistry 1957 224: 803-810
US Department of Justice, <u>DEA. CHADD and Ritalin</u>. 1995

van Praag, H.M. "Serotonin precursors in the treatment of depression." <u>Advanced Biochemical</u> <u>Psychopharmacol</u>. 1982: 34:259-86.
Vedantam, S. "Antidepressant Makers Withhold Data on Children." <u>Washington Post</u> 2004, Jan. 29: A01
Vedantam, S. "FDA Told Analyst to Censor Data on Antidepressants." <u>Washington Post</u> 2004, Sept. 24: A08

Walsh, K. & McDougle, C. "When SSRI's make sense for pediatric use." <u>Patient Care</u> 2002, Feb. 28: p. 25
Waters, Rob. "What Parents Aren't Being Told About Their Kid's Antidepressants-A Suicide Effect." <u>San Francisco Chronicle</u> Jan 10, 2004.
Werbach, M. <u>Nutritional Influences on Mental Illness</u>, Third Line Press, Tarzana, CA, Feb. 1999: p 128.
Willman, D. "A Federal Researcher Who Defended a Client's Lethal Drug." <u>Los Angeles Times</u> 2003, Dec. 7: 10A
Willman, D. "Stealth Merger: Drug Companies and Government Medical Research," <u>Los Angeles Times</u> 2003, Dec. 7.
Willman, D. "NIH Is Pressured to Bar Drug Industry Stipends." <u>Los Angeles Times</u> 2004, Aug. 6.
Wilson, Robert A. <u>Feminine Forever</u>, Evans and Company, 1966
<u>Women's Health Initiative</u> . July 17, 2002.

Young, A. & Adams, C. "Off-label Drugs Take Their Toll." <u>Knight-Ridder Newspapers</u> 2003, Nov. 2.

Young, A. & Adams, C. "Drug Makers' Promotions Boost Off-label Use by Doctors." <u>Knight-Ridder Newspapers</u> 2003, Nov. 3.

Young, A. & Adams, C. "FDA Oversight of 'Off-label' Drug Use Wanes." <u>Knight-Ridder Newspapers</u> 2003, Nov. 4.

Young, A. & Adams, C. "Samples Pave Way for Rxes." <u>Knight-Ridder Newspapers</u> 2003, Nov. 6.

Zuckerman, G. "Biovail Pushes Drug Aggressively." <u>Wall Street Journal</u> 2003, Jul. 21: C7

INDEX

ADHD (see Attention Deficit Hyperactivity Disorder)
adrenal gland, 69
allergies, 97-100
    depression and, 97
    testing and, 99-100
American Psychiatric Association
    definition of depression 11-12
antidepressants
    antihistamines and, 97
    children and, 44, 45, 46
    rate of prescriptions, 9, 45
    suicides and 44, 45-46
    withdrawal from, 107
Attention Deficit Hyperactivity Disorder (ADHD), 13-14
autism
    Cold Mother Syndrome, 13
    medical causes, 13-14

Bextra, viii
bipolar, 108-109

calcium, 86
Children and Adults with ADD (CHADD), 42
cortisone, 70-71
Cymbalta, 102

Dear Abby, 18-19
depression
    allergies and, 97
    Diagnostic and Statistical Manual and, 27-28
    genetics and, 19-20
    natural physical response, 17-18
    nutrient deficiency and, 89-90, 91-92
    physical illness and, 22, 23, 28
    screening and, 21
diagnosis, differential 24
Diagnostic and Statistical Manual
    conflict of interest and, 29

depression definition, 27-28
mental disorder definition, 30
neurological, general medical conditions, 31
psychiatric diagnosis recommendation, 31
drug companies (see pharmaceutical industry)

Effexor, viii
effectiveness disputed, 45
estrogen (estrogen dominance), 75
bio-identical forms of, 79-80
replacement therapy, 77-79

Food and Drug Administration (FDA)
antidepressant warning labels and, 45
drug approval process, 36-37
government protection of, 44
off-label prescriptions and, 50
pharmaceutical industry influence and, 50-51
Rezulin and, 36-37
Rotavirus vaccine and, 36
SSRIs and, 47, 50-53
thalidomide and, 50

Health Maintenance Organization (HMO), viii, 55
HMO (see Health Maintenance Organization)
hormones (female)
bio-identical, 8, 76
imbalances, effects of, 8, 68, 69
medical research and, 77
replacement therapy and, 77-79
hyperthyroidism, 63
hypothyroidism, 25
Diagnostic and Statistical Manual and, 30
individual experiences with, 25, 30, 61-62
insurance companies and, 67-68
symptoms, 68
informed consent, 24, 104-105
insurance industry
drug-based medicine and, 56
influence on medical care, 53-56

psychiatric diagnosis and, 29, 61-62
iodine 62

Lexapro, viii

magnesium, 86, 89-91
        deficiency, 89-90, 91
        depletion of, 90
        supplements, 89
medical errors, 106
menopause, 74
mental health parity, 14
mental illness
        definition, 11

National Institute of Health, 37-38
        clinical trials and, 49
Neurontin, viii
neurotransmitters, 17, 93-94

off-label prescriptions, 49-53
        federal law and, 52
        individual experiences and, 51
        value of, 52

Paxil, viii
        children and (Britain), 48
        clinical trials and, 48-49
        indiviudal experiences and, 46
        suicide risk and, 44-45, 47
PDR (see Physicians Desk Reference)
pharmaceutical industry
        defense of SSRIs, 47-49
        drug approval process, 36-37
        drug testing process, 37-40, 47-48
        free samples and, 52-53
        government protection and, 44, 49-50
        influence on doctors, 34-37, 48-49
        influence on consumers, 42-44
        influence on research 36-37

National Institute of Health and, 37-38
new drugs, profitability of, 40-41
patents and, 41-42
Phentermine, viii
Phillips, Jeanne (See Dear Abby)
Physicians Desk Reference (PDR), 7
Pitan, Brad, 102-104
PMDD (see Premenstrual Dysphoric Disorder)
post-partum depression, 9, 19
    individual experiences with, 73
    public debate and, 84
Premarin, 75, 77
    adverse effects and, 78-79
    calcium interaction and, 86
Premenstrual Dysphoric Disorder (PMDD), 9, 84-85
    Sarafem and, 41, 84-85
    symptoms and, 84, 85
Premenstrual Syndrome (PMS), 74
progesterone, 75-76, 77, 80
Provigil, 52-53
Provera, 77
Prozac
    effectiveness disputed, 45
    individual experiences with, 3-8, 56, 61
    patent and, 41-42
    re-marketed as Sarafem, 41
psychiatric diagnoses
    chemical imbalances, 18
    Diagnostic and Statistical Manual recommendation, 30-31
    individual experiences with, 33-34
    insurance industry and, 29
    physical exams and, 16
    potential underlying conditions, 25, 28

Risperdal, 51, 52
Ritalin, 15
    individual experiences with, 15, 61-62

Selective Serotonin Reuptake Inhibitors (SSRI)
    cancer risk with, 9-10

children and, 107-108
FDA hearings and, 45-46
FDA warnings and, 44
Great Britain, banned in, 43-44
individual experiences with, 45-46, 51
pharmaceutical industry and, 46-48, 94-95
risks and, 44-51, 104-105
sales of, 49
serotonin
5-HTP and, 92
depletion of, 92-93
Sarafem (see Prozac)
SSRI (see Selective Serotonin Reuptake Inhibitors)

TeenScreen, 14
Terbutaline, 51
thalidomide, 49
multiple myeloma treatment and, 50
thyroid (see also hyperthyroidism, hypothyroidism)
function of, 62
imbalances, effects of, 9
pharmaceutical industry and, 68-69
replacement therapy, 8, 69
testing procedures, 65-67
TSH (thyroid stimulating hormone), 9, 68
Topamax, 51
tricyclic antidepressants, 97

Vioxx, viii

Wellbutrin, viii

Xanax, viii
Yates, Andrea, 81-84

Zoloft, viii
individual experiences with, 8-9, 45-46, 102-104
effectiveness disputed, 45
Zyprexa, 101-102, 108

Just Because You're Depressed